Portland Community College

Facilitating Aging in Place: Safe, Sound, and Secure

Editors

LAZELLE E. BENEFIELD
BARBARA J. HOLTZCLAW

NURSING CLINICS
OF NORTH AMERICA

www.nursing.theclinics.com

Consulting Editor
STEPHEN D. KRAU

June 2014 • Volume 49 • Number 2

ELSEVIER

1600 John F. Kennedy Boulevard • Suite 1800 • Philadelphia, Pennsylvania, 19103-2899

http://www.theclinics.com

NURSING CLINICS OF NORTH AMERICA Volume 49, Number 2
June 2014 ISSN 0029-6465, ISBN-13: 978-0-323-29925-1

Editor: Kerry Holland
Developmental Editor: Casey Jackson

Nursing Clinics of North America (ISSN 0029-6465) is published quarterly by Elsevier Inc., 360 Park Avenue South, New York, NY 10010-1710. Months of issue are March, June, September, and December. Periodicals postage paid at New York, NY and additional mailing offices. Subscription price per year is, $150.00 (US individuals), $400.00 (US institutions), $275.00 (international individuals), $488.00 (international institutions), $220.00 (Canadian individuals), $488.00 (Canadian institutions), $85.00 (US students), and $135.00 (international students). To receive student/resident rate, orders must be accompanied by name of affiliated institution, date of term, and the signature of program/residency coordinator on institution letterhead. Orders will be billed at individual rate until proof of status is received. Foreign air speed delivery is included in all *Clinics* subscription prices. All prices are subject to change without notice. **POSTMASTER:** Send address changes to *Nursing Clinics*, Elsevier Health Sciences Division, Subscription Customer Service, 3251 Riverport Lane, Maryland Heights, MO 63043. **Customer Service: Telephone: 1-800-654-2452** (U.S. and Canada); **1-314-447-8871 (outside U.S. and Canada). Fax: 1-314-447-8029. E-mail: journalscustomerservice-usa@elsevier.com** (for print support) and **journalsonlinesupport-usa@elsevier.com** (for online support).

Nursing Clinics of North America is covered in *EMBASE/Excerpta Medica, MEDLINE/PubMed (Index Medicus), Social Sciences Citation Index, Current Contents, ASCA, Cumulative Index to Nursing, RNdex Top 100,* and Allied Health Literature and International Nursing Index (INI).

Printed in the United States of America.

Contributors

CONSULTING EDITOR

STEPHEN D. KRAU, PhD, RN, CNE
Associate Professor, Vanderbilt School of Nursing, Vanderbilt University Medical Center, Nashville, Tennessee

EDITORS

LAZELLE E. BENEFIELD, PhD, RN, FAAN
Parry Endowed Professor; Director, Donald W. Reynolds Center of Geriatric Nursing Excellence; Dean, University of Oklahoma Health Sciences Center College of Nursing, Oklahoma City, Oklahoma

BARBARA J. HOLTZCLAW, PhD, RN, FAAN
Associate Dean for Research; Associate Director of Geriatric Nursing Translational Research Training, Donald W. Reynolds Center of Geriatric Nursing Excellence, University of Oklahoma Health Sciences Center College of Nursing, Oklahoma City, Oklahoma

AUTHORS

ANNE ALGER, BSN, RN
Staff Nurse, Cardiac Care, OU Medical Center, Oklahoma City, Oklahoma

LAZELLE E. BENEFIELD, PhD, RN, FAAN
Parry Endowed Professor; Director, Donald W. Reynolds Center of Geriatric Nursing Excellence; Dean, University of Oklahoma Health Sciences Center College of Nursing, Oklahoma City, Oklahoma

KATHLEEN C. BUCKWALTER, PhD, RN, FAAN
Professor of Research & Distinguished Nurse Scientist in Aging, Donald W. Reynolds Center of Geriatric Nursing Excellence, Oklahoma University Health Sciences Center, Oklahoma City, Oklahoma

SANDY BURGENER, PhD, RN, FAAN
Associate Professor Emerita, University of Illinois College of Nursing, Urbana, Illinois

BARBARA W. CARLSON, PhD, RN
Professor, Donald W. Reynolds Center of Geriatric Nursing Excellence, The University of Oklahoma Health Sciences Center College of Nursing, Oklahoma City, Oklahoma

CARRIE A. CIRO, PhD, OTR/L, FAOTA
Assistant Professor, Department of Rehabilitation Sciences, University of Oklahoma Health Sciences Center, Oklahoma City, Oklahoma

MARIA CORDEIRO, MS, APRN, CNP
PhD Student; Department of Nursing, Reynolds Center of Geriatric Nursing Excellence, University of Oklahoma Health Sciences Center College of Nursing, Oklahoma City, Oklahoma

MELISSA CRAFT, PhD, APRN, CNS, AOCN
Assistant Professor, University of Oklahoma Health Sciences Center College of Nursing, Oklahoma City, Oklahoma

ELENA CUADERES, PhD, RN
Associate Professor, University of Oklahoma Health Sciences Center College of Nursing, Oklahoma City, Oklahoma

KATHY HENLEY HAUGH, PhD, RN, CNE
Assistant Professor, University of Virginia School of Nursing, Charlottesville, Virginia

BARBARA J. HOLTZCLAW, PhD, RN, FAAN
Associate Dean for Research; Associate Director of Geriatric Nursing Translational Research Training, Donald W. Reynolds Center of Geriatric Nursing Excellence, University of Oklahoma Health Sciences Center College of Nursing, Oklahoma City, Oklahoma

KIMETHRIA L. JACKSON, RN, MSN, FNP, APRN
The Substance Abuse and Mental Health Services Administration and the American Nurse Association Minority Fellowship Program Fellow 2013-2014; Donald W. Reynolds Predoctoral Scholar 2011-2013, Donald W. Reynolds Center of Geriatric Nursing Excellence, University of Oklahoma Health Sciences Center College of Nursing, Oklahoma City, Oklahoma

RACHEL KLIMMEK, PhD, RN
Department of Community and Public Health, School of Nursing, Johns Hopkins University, Baltimore, Maryland

W. LYNDON LAMB, DPM
Podiatrist, Podiatry, Choctaw Nation Health Care Center, Talihina, Oklahoma

MANKA NKIMBENG, MPH, BSN
Department of Community and Public Health, School of Nursing, Johns Hopkins University, Baltimore, Maryland

MARY H. PALMER, PhD, RN, C FAAN, AGSF
Professor, Division of Adult and Geriatric Health, School of Nursing; Helen W. & Thomas L. Umphlet Distinguished Professor in Aging Interim; Co-Director Institute on Aging, The University of North Carolina at Chapel Hill, Chapel Hill, North Carolina

ERICA PERRYMAN, BBA
Research Assistant, Department of Nursing, Reynolds Center of Geriatric Nursing Excellence, University of Oklahoma Health Sciences Center College of Nursing, Oklahoma City, Oklahoma

REBECCA J. RILEY, MSW, PhD
Adjunct Faculty, Department of Gerontology, University of Nebraska at Omaha, Omaha, Nebraska

CAROL E. ROGERS, PhD, RN
Assistant Professor, Department of Nursing, Donald W Reynolds Center of Geriatric Nursing Excellence, University of Oklahoma Health Sciences Center College of Nursing, Oklahoma City, Oklahoma

JILL ROTH, BSN
Department of Community and Public Health, School of Nursing, Johns Hopkins University, Baltimore, Maryland

JESSICA SAVAGE, BSN
Department of Community and Public Health, School of Nursing, Johns Hopkins University, Baltimore, Maryland

JANET SULLIVAN-WILSON, PhD, RN
Associate Professor; Associate Director, Donald W. Reynolds Center of Geriatric Nursing Excellence Community Based Interdisciplinary Research, University of Oklahoma Health Sciences Center College of Nursing, Oklahoma City, Oklahoma

SARAH L. SZANTON, PhD, ANP
Associate Professor, Department of Community and Public Health, School of Nursing, Johns Hopkins University, Baltimore, Maryland

Contents

> Barriers to aging in place include physical mobility and transportation lim- itations, isolation related loneliness and depression, diminishing health status, housing quality, finances, and caregiving resources. The scope of the aging demographic shift, economic consequences and loss of quality of life urge adoption of such successful approaches as the life course model. Desirable aging in place provides person-centered quality of living that is independence-effective and affordable. Systematic community-centered and person-centered approaches are crucial to accomplishing the central actions of the life course model. Not only are the actions necessary, they are interactive, interdependent, and strategic in supporting one another.

> Aging with independence benefits individuals, family, and society. To achieve independence, older adults must be able to function in their homes. This function is determined both by their abilities and by the environment in which they maneuver. This article describes a promising program that intervenes with both older adults and their home environ- ments to improve function. This program, called CAPABLE (Community Aging in Place, Advancing Better Living for Elders), is funded through the Affordable Care Act and can be scaled up nationally if determined to be a success in improving health and decreasing health care costs.

> Inactivity leads to frailty and loss of function for older adults. Most older adults are sedentary. Participating in a regular routine of physical activity is recommended for maintaining physical function required to sustain qual- ity of life and independence for older adults. Annual screening for level of physical activity is required to determine changes from year to year. Re- search shows older adults are more likely to initiate a regular routine of physical activity when a health care provider writes a prescription for phys- ical activity including the type, frequency, and specific duration of physical activity sessions.

and may result in anxiety in persons with dementia. This article focuses on anxiety, one of the least understood symptoms associated with dementia in community-dwelling older adults, the stigma of dementia, and the relationship between anxiety and stigma in dementia. When undetected and untreated, anxiety and associated stigma can adversely affect quality of life and the ability to age in place.

Nocturia is a bothersome symptom that increases with age, resulting in sleep disruption, an increased risk of falls, and a greater likelihood of rating one's health as poor. It is often a symptom of conditions that cause low volume voiding, overproduction of urine across the day or only at night and a symptom of a sleep disorder. Nocturia affects quality of life and has an impact on aging in place, thus assessment and treatment are essential. Behavioral treatments should be explored first, keeping in mind what the affected older adult defines as the desired outcomes of treatment.

Making individual recommendations for cancer screening in older adult patients may be difficult and time consuming, because of the need to incorporate complex issues of life expectancy, health status, risks and benefits, and individual values and wishes. In this article, current recommendations and related risks and benefits are summarized. Specific issues and concerns are addressed, with suggestions for strategies to assist older adults in making screening decisions.

NURSING CLINICS OF NORTH AMERICA

DOWNLOAD
Free App!

Review Articles
THE CLINICS

NOW AVAILABLE FOR YOUR iPhone and iPad

Foreword

Meeting the Challenges of Aging and Health-related Changes

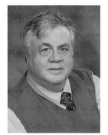

Stephen D. Krau, PhD, RN, CNE
Consulting Editor

Grow old along with me!

The best is yet to be,

The last of life, for which the first was made.
　　　　　　　—*Robert Browning, From "Rabbi Ben Ezra"*

In view of the anticipated continued growth in home and community-based services (HCBS), care for the elderly will likely experience a corresponding increase in the demand for nursing and health care resources. New models for caring for the elderly are warranted to meet the challenges for nurses, nursing educational programs, as well as policymakers and employers of registered nurses. The 2010 Affordable Care Act, as well as prior efforts at health care reform, has provided a portal for attention to innovations in care for all persons including elderly in long-term care, ambulatory care, as well as home services and community-based services.[1]

The complexity associated with the number of persons born during the "Baby Boom," along with the fact that people are living longer with chronic illnesses and the growing arena of treatments and medications, makes traditional perspectives in caring for the elderly obsolete. Current health care reform provisions focus on reducing health care expenditures, especially when considering the growing population of older adults.[1] Health care policymakers now know what health care providers have expressed for many years, that it is more cost-effective to care for individuals in their homes, and communities, rather than institutions, while at the same time preserving individual preferences to live independently in their homes as long as possible.

The AARP Public Policy Institute published the results of an extensive study examining the actual or potential fiscal impact (or justification) of HCBS as alternatives to

Nurs Clin N Am 49 (2014) xi–xii
http://dx.doi.org/10.1016/j.cnur.2014.04.001
0029-6465/14/$ – see front matter © 2014 Published by Elsevier Inc.

nursing facility care.[2] Although few studies that were considered in this mega-analysis document absolute cost-savings, the studies consistently found much lower per-individual, average costs for HCBS compared with care in an institution. Overall, the results identified significant cost reductions by diverting and transitioning individuals from nursing home care to HCBS.[2] For example, in California, HCBS spending was one-third ($9129) the cost of nursing facility care ($32,406) in 2008.[2]

Aging in place not only has financial benefits to the individual and the health care system as a whole but also demonstrates implied benefits as well. This is exemplified in the findings of a study examining Emergency Department (ED) visits for persons living in a nursing care facility. Nursing home residents have a disproportionately higher rate of ED visits, many of which are preventable, when compared with all Americans over the age of 65. When considering specific potentially preventable ambulatory care–sensitive conditions, the ED visits for nursing home residents in 2007 was 1310 visits per 1000, as compared with all Americans over 65, where the rate was 476.8 visits per 1000.[3]

Issues related to aging, and living in the home, transcend basic health care issues. In addition, communities, attitudes, and services for the elderly demand reconsideration and intercession. This involves the creation of new models to keep the elderly engaged in our society as well as new approaches to involve multiple disciplines, multiple agencies, and more intentional public education. *Life course theory* offers a perspective that has been used for decades by social scientists to explore people's lives within structural, social, and cultural contexts.[4] Interprofessional, interdisciplinary, and legislative awareness and the perspective offered through the lens of the complete life course present an approach to meet many of the challenges of aging and the elderly.

Stephen D. Krau, PhD, RN, CNE
Vanderbilt School of Nursing
Vanderbilt University Medical Center
461 21st Avenue, South
Nashville, TN 37240, USA

E-mail address:
steve.krau@vanderbilt.edu

REFERENCES

1. Rosenfeld P, Russell D. A review of factors influencing utilization of home and community-based long-term care: trends and implications to the nursing workforce. Policy Polit Nurs Pract 2012;13(2):72–80.
2. AARP Public Policy Institute. State studies find home and community based services to be cost effective. March 2013. Available at: http://www.aarp.org/health/medicare-insurance/info-03-2013/state-studies-find-hcbs-to-be-cost-effective-AARP-ppi-ltc.html. Accessed April 6, 2014.
3. Brownell BA, Wang J, Smith A, et al. Trends in emergency department visits for ambulatory care sensitive conditions by elderly nursing home residents, 2001-2010. JAMA Intern Med 2014;174(1):156–8.
4. Mayer KU. New directions in life course research. Annu Rev Sociol 2009;35:413–33.

Preface

Aging in Place: A Life Course Perspective

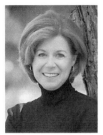
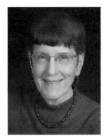

Lazelle E. Benefield, PhD, RN, FAAN   Barbara J. Holtzclaw, PhD, RN, FAAN
Editors

INTRODUCTION

Aging in place, whereby older adults remain at home or a similar preferred setting for as long as possible with as much ability and dignity as possible, involves addressing health- and age-related changes within a coordinated plan of health care, social, financial, hous- ing, technology, and resource use. The need to consider issues surrounding health care in an aging population is painfully urgent. Challenges to older adults for dealing with longer life, declining health, and fewer resources are highly complex. Seeking ap- proaches that facilitate aging in place poses challenges beyond health care and no generic plan can adequately meet every older adult's needs. An integrative approach, viewing problems and solutions from a *life course* perspective makes sense on several levels. Derived from *life course theory*, the approach has been used by social scientists for decades to analyze people's lives within structural, social, and cultural contexts.[1] The need for solutions to promote and maintain health, offer social support, and assure safe environments calls for interprofessional and cross-disciplinary collaboration.

The idyllic dreams of restful recreation, vacation travel, or visits to relatives are often economically or physically impossible. Planning for the future for many adults has been inadequate, based on unrealistic expectations of what advanced age would actually be like. Many older persons reside in residences not fully supportive of their life stage needs. Most homes fall into the category of "Peter Pan housing," quips Dr Jon Pynoos, professor at USC Davis School of Gerontology. The term refers to houses designed for persons who are never going to age and consequently are plagued with obstacles in three major areas: getting in and out of the house, up and down stairs, and using the bathroom.[2] Home infrastructure deteriorates over time[3] and is compounded by physical demands associated with home maintenance[4] and increases in property taxes and utility costs.[5] Limited or no access to transportation due to the built

Nurs Clin N Am 49 (2014) xiii–xv
http://dx.doi.org/10.1016/j.cnur.2014.02.011
0029-6465/14/$ – see front matter © 2014 Elsevier Inc. All rights reserved.

community environment may limit the older adults' daily functioning while available transportation may be unusable due to concerns about public transit's safety, personal security, flexibility, reliability, and comfort.[6]

Aging in place has been made more complex by scientific advances that have maintained life and cured illnesses while increasing numbers of older adults with longer life spans. However, declining health, increasing costs for health care, lower capacity for self-care, and higher risks for age-related comorbidities are often unwelcome correlates of growing older in a poor economy. In short, longer lives can often mean more years of poor health and dependency for many. As a result, the gap between environmental accommodations and realistic individual expectations widens. There is urgency for nursing to engage with interdisciplinary colleagues to help older adults not simply live longer, but live healthier lives with less disability. By combining expertise and experience to translate science and inform a common care concern, interaction across disciplines often leads to better health-promoting outcomes to postpone institutionalization of older adults with physical and cognitive impairments.

The articles appearing in this geriatrics-focused issue of *Nursing Clinics of North America* are consistent with the collaborative and translational concepts held by a life course perspective. Each supports interprofessional collaboration and some are either authored or coauthored by interdisciplinary colleagues. Three goals are reflected in these articles: keeping community-dwelling older adults safe, sensible, and secure with solutions that will enable them to stay healthy, wise, and aware. Topics include maintaining physical functions, benefits and consequences of weight-bearing exercise on foot health; cancer prevention; managing nocturia's effect on sleep quality and safety, protection from financial exploitation, and providing safe and affordable living environments. Several articles address physical or cognitive challenges that include monitoring medication adherence, threat of anxiety and stigma in dementia, and approaches to managing self-care in the home for persons with dementia. These evidence-based articles address emerging and best practices to support targeted interventions for persons in community-dwelling home settings. They provide a framework of person-centered approaches that foster good health in older age, a central tenet of aging in place and the global response to population aging.[7]

Lazelle E. Benefield, PhD, RN, FAAN
University of Oklahoma Health Sciences Center
College of Nursing
1100 North Stonewall
Oklahoma City, OK 73117, USA

Barbara J. Holtzclaw, PhD, RN, FAAN
University of Oklahoma Health Sciences Center
College of Nursing
1100 North Stonewall
Oklahoma City, OK 73117, USA

E-mail addresses:
Lazelle-Benefield@ouhsc.edu (L.E. Benefield)
Barbara-Holtzclaw@ouhsc.edu (B.J. Holtzclaw)

REFERENCES

1. Mayer KU. New directions in life course research. Ann Rev Sociol 2009;35: 413–33.

2. Bezatitis A. New technologies for aging in place. Aging Well 2008;1(2):26.
3. Scharlach AE. Frameworks for fostering aging-friendly community change: recent local, regional, national, and transnational initiatives. Generations 2009;33(2): 71–3.
4. Pynoos J, Caraviello R, Cicero C. Lifelong housing: the anchor in aging-friendly communities. Generations 2009;33(2):26–32.
5. Sabia JJ. There's no place like home: a hazard model analysis of aging in place among older homeowners in the PSID. Res Aging 2008;30(1):3–35.
6. Rosenbloom S. Meeting transportation needs in an aging-friendly community: surprisingly, the most promising focus may be on keeping older people driving longer. Generations 2009;33(2):33–43.
7. WHO. Good health adds life to years: global brief for World Health Day 2012. Geneva (Switzerland): World Health Organization. Available at: http://whqlibdoc.who.int/hq/2012/WHO_DCO_WHD_2012.2_eng.pdf?ua=1. Accessed July 12, 2012.

Aging in Place
Merging Desire with Reality

Lazelle E. Benefield, PhD, RN, FAAN*, Barbara J. Holtzclaw, PhD, RN, FAAN

KEYWORDS

- Aging in place • Older adults • Person-centered care • Life course perspective
- Interdisciplinary • Gerontechnology • Care coordination

KEY POINTS

- There is urgency for nursing to engage with interdisciplinary colleagues to help older adults not simply live longer, but live healthier lives with less disability.
- Aging in place, whereby older adults remain at home or a similar preferred setting for as long as possible with as much ability and dignity as possible, involves addressing health-related and age-related changes within a coordinated plan of health care, social, financial, housing, technology, and resource use.
- In the best of circumstances, aging in place represents a physical and social environmental model, enabling older adults to stay connected, maintain dignity, pride, independence, and autonomy, and maximize financial resources.
- The challenge, therefore, is addressing the wide variety of living arrangements matched to the older adult's present and future function to predict a trajectory of care.
- To create successful aging in place, community as well as family/person support are required.

INTRODUCTION
Aging in Place Defined

The Centers for Disease Control and Prevention define aging in place as "the ability to live in one's own home and community safely, independently, and comfortably, regardless of age, income, or ability level,"[1] From a life course perspective, aging in place is a situation whereby older adults remain at home or a similar preferred setting for as long as possible with as much ability and dignity as possible. It involves addressing health-related and age-related changes within a coordinated plan of health care with social, financial, housing, technology, and resource considerations. Surveys

Funding Sources: This work was supported by a grant from the Donald W. Reynolds Foundation. Conflict of Interest: None.
Donald W. Reynolds Center of Geriatric Nursing Excellence, University of Oklahoma Health Sciences Center College of Nursing, 1100 North Stonewall, Oklahoma City, OK 73117, USA
* Corresponding author.
E-mail address: Lazelle-Benefield@ouhsc.edu

of US adults show that more than 90% of 65-year-olds to 74-year-olds and 95% of those older than 75 years, who are living in single-family detached homes, wish to remain there as long as possible.[2,3] Place is therefore a broad and complex conceptual matrix, embracing both the physical and the social environment. Its psychological component has a distinctive meaning for each person.[4] Stereotypes of older adults living among friendly community and family supports fail to represent the situations of many, and increase of the aging population drives an imperative for serious advanced planning.

Aging in place independently, in a safe, comfortable environment of one's choice, is philosophically attractive, whether it refers to one's home, community dwellings, or a special facility. However, the idyllic dreams of restful recreation, vacation travel, or visits to relatives are often economically or physically impossible. In reality, there are issues that challenge an aging adult's safety, health, and economic security beyond the choice of location. Numerous intrinsic and extrinsic factors threaten possibilities for safe and sound health in the residence of one's choice. Disparities exist between the older adult's desire to live independently, realities of declining health and function, and the financial ability to secure adequate housing. Seeking approaches that facilitate aging in place logically poses challenges beyond health care. Social scientists, adult protective organizations, and governmental agencies began addressing the increasing populations of older adults as a major challenge of the millennium.[2] Surveys of older adults document that poor health, low quality of life, and loss of mobility that accompany late life must refocus efforts beyond just increasing life span to goals of increasing health span.[5] The need for solutions to promote and maintain health, offer social support, and ensure safe environments calls for interprofessional and cross-disciplinary collaboration and a perspective that encompasses these factors. Along with interdisciplinary involvement, there is need for a unifying perspective to conceptualize the myriad of issues confronting aging in place. There is growing evidence that a model viewing aging in place within a life course perspective is particularly well suited to this task.[6–8] This approach has been used by social scientists for decades to analyze people's lives within structural, social, and cultural contexts, with balanced effort in each of these areas.[8] In applying these principles to aging in place, these 4 key tenets are addressed: (1) consumer/older person decision making, (2) technology as a core support structure, (3) interdisciplinary focus, and (4) placement of care coordination as a proven method of intervention.

REALITIES OF AGING ENVIRONMENTS

Many older persons reside in home environments not particularly suited to social, safe, mobile, and active aging. Many determinants of health and active aging are beyond the influence of the health system and include family caregiver support, adequate financial resources, access to social and community resources, and safe neighborhoods. Many older persons reside in home settings not fully supportive of their life stage needs. Most houses have been designed for persons who are never going to age, with obstacles in 3 major areas: getting in and out of the house, up and down stairs, and using the bathroom.[9] Home infrastructure deterioration occurs over time and is compounded by physical demands associated with maintaining a home and increases in property taxes and usefulness costs.[10–12] Limited or no access to transportation because of the built community environment may limit the older adult's daily functioning. Available transportation may be unusable because of concerns about safety, personal security, flexibility, reliability, and comfort in public transit.[13]

Changes in family composition also pose challenges to aging in place. Older adults serve roles in the family structure, which are affected by diminished physical or social well-being.[12] Demographics and family locations change, leaving fewer older persons with family support.[14] By choice or economics, older adults or their children may live at a distance, and general family interactions and family member caregiving becomes more challenging than onsite or nearby caregiving. Those older adults who feel compelled to stay in their existing home, because of financial constraints or social reasons, can experience mounting levels of loneliness, helplessness, and boredom.[15] Therefore, for some, aging in place is neither a choice nor a viable option. Aging in place within a home setting may be unappealing even with full function; severe physical disability or dementia may require supportive care that is better provided in other care settings. The challenge, therefore, is to address living arrangements that are matched to the older adult's present and future function to predict a trajectory of care. However, we believe that attention to the trajectory of ever-changing needs should be considered a tenet of aging in place.

LOCAL CRISES IN A GLOBAL CONTEXT

Accurately predicting this trajectory is highly variable, and not within the scope of this article. Communities in the United States have not been entirely responsive to the realities that aging and chronic illness present to older adults with comorbid health conditions. Older adults find that they have not planned realistic living arrangements, transportation means, social links, or recreation for later life. Even when finances are adequate, older adults with disabilities cannot always find accommodation or transportation near families or friends. Senior living communities are often equipped for the newly retired active adult who still drives an automobile. As a result, the gap between available environmental accommodations and realistic individual expectations widens. It is not surprising that those who had expected more satisfaction, relaxation, and social interaction in later life find the disparity disappointing.[15]

The dichotomy between desire and reality are equally present in the older adult's search for appropriate health care, as families and aging adults deal with a system still geared toward cure and survival to prolong life. Aging in place consequently has become more complex by scientific advances that lengthen life for those with chronic disease. Although people age, declining health, increasing costs for health care, lower capacity for self-care, and higher risks for age-related comorbidities are frequently unwelcome correlates of growing older in a poor economy. Increasing annual readmission rates in emergency departments and hospitals attest to the frequency with which the system temporarily navigates older adults through distressing acute care crisis treatments, only to discharge them to settings unable to manage the predisposing condition. Longer lives can often mean more years of poor health and dependency. Paradoxically, the younger population, on whom the aging expect to depend, grows smaller in proportion. For the first time in history, the global aging population of adults older than 65 years will soon outnumber young children.[14]

Improving health span by living well within one's capabilities is a global challenge to population aging.[5] The World Health Organization (WHO) makes it clear that outliving one's health is not a problem unique to the United States in their emphasis on population aging as a transforming demographic force. In their 2012 Global Brief, *Good Health Adds Life to Years*,[5] WHO's recommendations in "A life-course approach to healthy and active aging"[5(p7)] go beyond physical requirements of the aging population, to include needs for changing social attitudes to build a society in which older people are respected and valued (**Fig. 1**).[16] The approach includes: (1) "Promoting

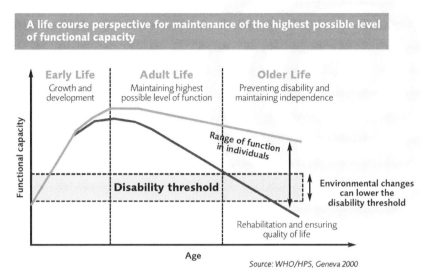

Fig. 1. WHO 2000 report: a life course approach to health and active aging. (*From* World Health Organization (WHO). The implications for training of embracing: A life course approach to health. Geneva (Switzerland): World Health Organization; 2000.)

good health and healthy behaviors at all ages to prevent or delay the development of chronic diseases"... (2) "Minimizing the consequences of chronic disease through early detection and quality care (primary, long-term and palliative care")... (3) "Creating physical and social environments that foster the health and participation of older people"... (4) "Reinventing ageing–changing social attitudes to encourage the participation of older people."[5(p7)]

There is a growing urgency for nursing to engage interdisciplinary colleagues and community partners to assist older adults; not to simply live longer, but to live healthier lives with less disability. Interaction across disciplines combines expertise and experience to translate science and inform a common care concern. These combined efforts arrive at person-centered approaches that foster good health in older age. The unifying life span perspective provides a framework across disciplines that is supportive of the central tenets of local and global approaches to aging in place.

LIFE COURSE PERSPECTIVE TO ADDRESS PERSON-CENTERED REALITIES
Principles and Key Actions

A model of aging in place within a life course perspective draws on several principles that are consistent with life course theory of structural, social, and cultural contexts. Central actions that facilitate aging in place include: (1) inclusion of consumer/older person decision making, (2) technology as a core support structure, (3) interdisciplinary involvement, and (4) placement of care coordination as a proven method of intervention. Investing in these key actions aims at increasing health span, or healthful years, versus increasing life span with disability. Actions to foster relative health, independence, and dignity are sustained for as long as possible within one's life, whereas the percentage of time during which a person experiences disability, loss of function, and dependence is reduced (**Fig. 2**).[17,18] In the best of circumstances, aging in place represents a physical and social environmental model enabling older adults to stay

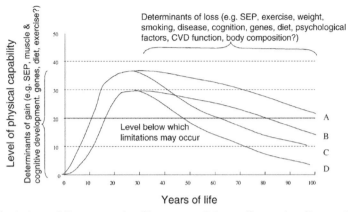

Fig. 2. Physical capability across the life course. CVD, cardiovascular disease; SEP, socio-economic position. (*From* Kuh D. A life course approach to healthy aging, frailty, and capability. J Gerontol A Biol Sci Med Sci 2007;62(7):718; with permission.)

connected, maintain dignity, pride, independence, and autonomy, and maximize financial resources.[19–22] Desirable aging in place provides person-centered quality of living that is independence effective[23] and affordable.[24] Desirable outcomes would likewise be measureable with such positive health measures as self-ratings of well-being, quality of life, maintenance of physical activity, and decreasing mortality risk and symptoms of depression.[25]

Implementing a Life Course Model

A systematic community-centered and person-centered approach is crucial to accomplishing the central actions of the life course model. Not only are the actions necessary, they are interactive, interdependent, and strategic in supporting one another.

INCLUSION OF THE CONSUMER/OLDER PERSON DECISION MAKING

To create successful aging in place, support from the community, the family, and the older adult is necessary. The traditional approach to where and how a person ages is typically based solely on overly simplified determinants of physical health. By contrast, a systematic approach includes attention to aging-friendly components of a community, physical environment of the home, and availability of family support and person-centered care. An aging-friendly community promotes both physical and psychosocial well-being of community members throughout the life cycle. As Scharlach's guest editorial in the *Journal of the American Society on Aging* aptly described it, "... a community might be considered aging-friendly to the extent that its major systems (housing, transportation/mobility, health, social interaction, productivity, cultural and religious involvement, educational and leisure activity) are responsive to the changing needs and capabilities of its members as they age, providing opportunities for fulfillment with regard to 5 psychosocial developmental tasks of later life: continuity, compensation, connection, contribution, and challenge."[10(p9)]

Family support and person-centered care are essential to sustaining independence at home, not only through social connectedness but also to maintain function and limit disability. Yet, this role is often overlooked. The term family is broadly defined here to include significant others within the household or social network, and person-centered care includes the well-known tenets of patient preference and responsiveness to needs and values.[26] The family is encouraged, with the older adult, to the extent possible, to use workable home-based interventions to maintain function in the 4 largest areas of disability: visual impairment, dementia, hearing loss, and osteoarthritis. Another focus of concern is in fall prevention. Physical injuries, particularly falls, often precipitate a progressive decline in function toward disability. Furthermore, family and communities can together engage in programs to prevent maltreatment and exploitation of the older adult; a situation that creates both physical and psychological consequences.[5]

TECHNOLOGY AS A CORE SUPPORT STRUCTURE

Systematic facilitators to aging in place incorporate methods and design features that support the living environment and the life activities of older adults. These factors include: (1) proper built environment, lighting, and railings; (2) sufficient social support, involving both social networks and social resources; and (3) supports to address potential health and safety concerns arising between the older adult, their environment, their own physical and mental well-being, and their links to others.[4,19,21,25,27,28] The intersection of aging and technology, termed gerontechnology, endorses and includes designing and use of technological environments to support changing life goals and lifestyle preferences of older persons across health, comfort, and safety.[29] Technology is used by providers (eg, remote telecare) and by older adults and family members to support aging in place in the living environment. Specific technology-based assistive devices include (1) supports to provide adaptation to physical, sensory, or cognitive decline, (2) monitor and response systems across emergency and routine function support, and (3) social communication aids. Technologies may be readily apparent or ubiquitous in the living environment, ranging from simple auto reminders to sophisticated cueing and online cognitive training.[30] Technology should serve an enabling role to support well-being and health.

INTERDISCIPLINARY INVOLVEMENT

Geriatrics and gerontology are interdisciplinary sciences derived from a variety of basic and biobehavioral fields. Disciplines that engage in this work include health-related fields of nursing, medicine, pharmacy, social work, physical and occupational therapy, and, but not limited to architecture, urban planning, law, engineering, and other technology professions. Understanding this diversity should remove any assumptions that all clinicians and health care practitioners in geriatric care share the same training, culture, values, language, and vision. These differences should be anticipated and strategically planned for.[31] Differing perspectives may provide more successful problem solving to address the complex issues associated with maintaining health span in one's living environment.

Well-organized team training is rare, with a few notable examples. The Veterans Administration Interdisciplinary Team Training was funded in 1995 "to improve the continuity and comprehensiveness of care for an aging veteran population," training more than 500 from nursing, social work, psychology, occupational therapy, pharmacy, dietetics, audiology, and speech pathology in interdisciplinary care.[32] Other support from federal government and philanthropic foundations for interdisciplinary programs in academic settings[33] has focused on key methods of organizing, training for, and implementing care within this model.

PLACEMENT OF CARE COORDINATION

A key tenet of the life course perspective is the use of care coordination as the method of delivery. It embraces proven cost-effective methods of aging in place care coordination by well-informed nurses. Care coordination appropriately occurs across transitions of care as well as during the continuum of care and changing care trajectories within the living environment. Although either care coordination or care navigation terms may be used, the framework includes an organized approach to delivering coordination services across health and social systems, including access to these and other community supports.[34]

Exemplary registered nurse care coordination with community facilitation within an aging in place model reveals cost-effectiveness and positive health measures compared with traditional long-term care.[23] Likewise, the Program of All-inclusive Care for the Elderly is widely known, and the program values participant function and capacity, preferences and goals, and care coordination with integrated intention and efficiency.[24] Certainly, although details cannot be included here, in both exemplars, the interdisciplinary team works in concert with the older person and family to identify key goals and outcomes.

SUMMARY

The model of aging in place presented here is framed by the life course perspective and centers on the following key tenets: person-centered in decision making, technology as a core assist, an interdisciplinary focus, and care coordination as the method of delivery. Barriers to aging in place include physical mobility limitations both in moving about the home and in transportation; loneliness and depression potentially caused by isolation; diminishing health status; economic hardships; poor housing quality; and lack of caregiving resources and support services.[35–38] These individual and community-based challenges are often not widely understood or viewed within a systems perspective.[14] There is also a lack of understanding of the scope of the aging demographic shift and resulting loss of quality of life and economic consequences of inaction. Although the adoption of successful aging in place models and interdisciplinary training have been historically slowed by limited data to support cost and health effectiveness beyond research trials, the need persists for both.

ACKNOWLEDGMENTS

Drs Benefield and Holtzclaw acknowledge the assistance of Erica Perryman, BBA, Research Assistant in the OU College of Nursing, in preparing this article.

REFERENCES

1. Centers for Disease Control (CDC). Healthy places terminology. Atlanta (GA): Centers for Disease Control; 2013. Available at: http://www.cdc.gov/healthyplaces/terminology.htm. Accessed October 13, 2013.
2. Jackson R, Howe N. Global aging: the challenge of the new millennium. AARP Ageline 2000. Available at: http://csis.org/files/media/csis/pubs/globalaging.pdf. Accessed October 13, 2013.
3. Mathew Greenwald. These four walls: Americans 45+ talk about home and community. 2003. Available at: http://www.aarp.org/content/dam/aarp/livable-communities/learn/housing/these-four-walls-americans-45plus-talk-about-home-and-community-aarp.pdf. Accessed October 13, 2013.

4. Chippendale TL, Bear-Lehman J. Enabling "aging in place" for urban dwelling seniors: an adaptive or remedial approach? Phys Occup Ther Geriatr 2010;28(1): 57–62.

5. World Health Organization (WHO). Good health adds life to years: global brief for World Health Day 2012. Available at: http://whqlibdoc.who.int/hq/2012/WHO_DCO_WHD_2012.2_eng.pdf. Accessed March 7, 2014.

6. Partners for Livable Communities. A blueprint for action: developing livable communities for all ages 2006. Available at: http://www.livable.org/livability-resources/reports-a-publications/184. Accessed March 7, 2014.

7. Dishman E. Inventing wellness systems for aging in place. Computer 2004. Available at: http://www.computer.org/csdl/mags/co/2004/05/r5034-abs.html. Accessed October 15, 2013.

8. Mayer KU. New directions in life course research. Annu Rev Sociol 2009;35: 413–33.

9. Bezatitis A. New technologies for aging in place. Aging Well 2008;1(2):26. Available at: http://todaysgeriatricmedicine.com/archive/spring08p26.shtml. Accessed March 7, 2014.

10. Scharlach AE. Creating aging-friendly communities: why America's cities and towns must become better places to grow old. Generations 2009;33(2):5–11.

11. Pynoos J, Caraviello R, Cicero C. Lifelong housing: the anchor in aging-friendly communities. Generations 2009;33(2):26–32.

12. Sabia JJ. There's no place like home: a hazard model analysis of aging in place among older homeowners in the PSID. Res Aging 2008;30(1):3–35.

13. Rosenbloom S. Meeting transportation needs in an aging-friendly community: surprisingly, the most promising focus may be on keeping older people driving longer. Generations 2009;33(2):33–43.

14. National Institutes of Health (NIH). Global health and aging. A report from the World Health Organization, National Institute on Aging, and National Institutes of Health. Washington DC: NIA (NIH); 2012.

15. Thomas WH, Blanchard JM. Moving beyond place: aging in community. Generations 2009;33(2):12–7.

16. World Health Organization (WHO). The implications for training of embracing: a life course approach to health. 2000. Available at: http://www.who.int/ageing/publications/lifecourse/alc_lifecourse_training_en.pdf. Accessed October 13, 2013.

17. Lai WF, Chan ZC. Beyond sole longevity: a social perspective on healthspan extension. Rejuvenation Res 2011;14(1):83–8.

18. Kuh D. A life course approach to healthy aging, frailty, and capability. J Gerontol A Biol Sci Med Sci 2007;62(7):717–21.

19. Moldow LG. Rethinking senior living models. Long-term living: for the continuing care professional. 2013. p. 26–8. Available at: http://webproxy.ouhsc.edu/login?url=http://search.ebscohost.com/login.aspx?direct=true&db=rzh&AN=2012077905&site=ehost-live. Accessed October 13, 2013.

20. Witsø AE, Vik K, Ytterhus B. Participation in older home care recipients: a value-based process. Act Adapt Aging 2012;36(4):297–316.

21. Young D. Automating the quest to age in place. Rehab Manag 2012;25(9):10–5.

22. Pastalan LA, Schwarz B. University-linked retirement communities: student visions of eldercare. J Hous Elderly 1994;11(1):1–178.

23. Rantz MJ, Phillips L, Aud M, et al. Evaluation of aging in place model with home care services and registered nurse care coordination in senior housing. Nurs Outlook 2011;59(1):37–46.

24. Chin Hansen J, Hewitt M. PACE provides a sense of belonging for elders. Generations 2012;36(1):37–43.
25. Tang F, Lee Y. Social support networks and expectations for aging in place and moving. Res Aging 2011;33(4):444–64.
26. Committee on Quality of Health Care in America and Institute of Medicine. Crossing the quality chasm: a new health system for the 21st century 2001. Available at: http://www.iom.edu/Reports/2001/Crossing-the-Quality-Chasm-A-New-Health-System-for-the-21st-Century.aspx#sthash.3VymYzHR.dpuf. Accessed October 13, 2013.
27. Keyes L, Rader C, Berger C. Creating communities: Atlanta's Lifelong Community initiative. Phys Occup Ther Geriatr 2011;29(1):59–74.
28. Castle NG, Ferguson JC, Schulz R. Aging-friendly health and long-term-care services: innovation in elders' homes, in ambulatory settings, in institutions. Generations 2009;33(2):44–50.
29. International Society of Gerontechnology. Available at: http://gerontechnology.info/index.php/journal/pages/view/isghome. Accessed November 8, 2013.
30. Horgas A, Abowd G. The impact of technology on living environments for older adults. In: Pew R, Van Hemel S, editors. Technology for adaptive aging. Washington, DC: The National Academies Press; 2004. p. 230.
31. Choi BC. Multidisciplinarity, interdisciplinarity, and transdisciplinarity in health research, services, education and policy: 3. Discipline, inter-discipline distance, and selection of discipline. Clin Invest Med 2008;31(1):E41–8.
32. Baldwin DC Jr. Some historical notes on interdisciplinary and interprofessional education and practice in health care in the USA. J Interprof Care 2007;21(S1):23–37.
33. Fulmer T, Hyer K, Flaherty E, et al. Geriatric interdisciplinary team training program evaluation results. J Aging Health 2005;17(4):443–70.
34. Craig C, Eby D, Whittington J. Care coordination model: better care at lower cost for people with multiple health and social needs. IHI Innovation Series. Cambridge (MA): Institute for Healthcare Improvement; 2011.
35. Yen IH, Anderson LA. Built environment and mobility of older adults: important policy and practice efforts. J Am Geriatr Soc 2012;60(5):951–6.
36. Haltiwanger EP, Underwood NS. Life after driving: a community-dwelling senior's experience. Phys Occup Ther Geriatr 2011;29(2):156–67.
37. Réébola CB, Jones B. Sympathetic devices: communication technologies for inclusion. Phys Occup Ther Geriatr 2011;29(1):44–58.
38. Dye CJ, Willoughby DF, Battisto DG. Advice from rural elders: what it takes to age in place. Educ Gerontol 2011;37(1):74–93.

FURTHER READINGS

MetLife Mature Market Institute. The MetLife Aging in place workbook: your home as a care setting. New York: MetLife Mature Market Institute; 2010. Available at: http://www.stanford.edu/dept/worklife/cgi-bin/drupal/sites/default/files/pdf/Workbook.pdf. Accessed March 7, 2014.
Rudolph L, Caplan J, Ben-Moshe K, et al. Health in all policies: a guide for state and local governments. Washington, DC, Oakland (CA): American Public Health Association and Public Health Institute; 2013. Available at: http://www.apha.org/NR/rdonlyres/882690FE-8ADD-49E0-8270-94C0ACD14F91/0/HealthinAllPoliciesGuide169pages.PDF.

Improving Unsafe Environments to Support Aging Independence with Limited Resources

Sarah L. Szanton, PhD, ANP*, Jill Roth, BSN,
Manka Nkimbeng, MPH, BSN, Jessica Savage, BSN,
Rachel Klimmek, PhD, RN

KEYWORDS

- Function • Older adults • Disability • Interprofessional

KEY POINTS

- Aging with independence benefits individuals, family, and society but can be hard to achieve.
- Function is determined by both the person and the environment in which they maneuver.
- This article describes a promising program that intervenes with both older adults and their home environments to improve function.
- This program, called CAPABLE (Community Aging in Place, Advancing Better Living for Elders), is funded through the Affordable Care Act and can be scaled up nationally if determined to be a success.

Aging with independence is important to older adults for multiple reasons: it affords better quality of life for older individuals and their families,[1] and is a foundational American value that, when achieved, saves resources for society to use in other ways. The number of older adults in the United States is projected to continue growing,[2] making it increasingly urgent to identify ways to support aging with independence. For many older adults, the challenges are socioeconomic.[3] However, for almost everyone, at every income level, aging brings functional challenges that can compromise independence. These functional challenges result from interactions between an individual's health and the surrounding environment. Low-income older adults face even greater challenges to independence because they have more comorbidities[3]; experience more functional limitations as a result[4,5]; and, by definition, have fewer resources to modify their home environments. This combination places them at even greater risk

The authors have no financial conflicts of interest to disclose.
Department of Community and Public Health, School of Nursing, Johns Hopkins University, 525 North Wolfe Street, Baltimore, MD 21205, USA
* Corresponding author.
E-mail address: sszanto1@jhu.edu

for reduced activity levels, social isolation, falls, and other adverse events. This article explains how unsafe environments affect older adults with functional limitations, and describes an interprofessional model of care, called CAPABLE (Community Aging in Place, Advancing Better Living for Elders), which addresses both individual and environmental aspects of aging with independence. This article also provides tools and lessons for use while implementing this innovative model of care within a community of urban-dwelling, low-income older adults with multiple functional limitations.

UNSAFE EXTERIOR ENVIRONMENTS POSE BARRIERS TO AGING WITH INDEPENDENCE

Every level of the environment supports or inhibits function and health.[6] From the neighborhood surrounding an older adult's home, to the steps leading up to their front doors, to the interior of the house and each room; all of these environments affect an older adult's ability to function well enough to age in place.

Neighborhood

The neighborhood of residence can affect health and safety in later life, particularly in urban settings where factors such as broken or littered sidewalks and busy streets, a lack of safe spaces to exercise, or the geography of gun violence and other threats[7–10] pose risks that keep some older adults indoors. Some neighborhoods also contain food deserts, meaning places lacking markets with ready supplies of produce and other options essential to a healthy diet. Unsafe neighborhoods not only prevent older adults from engaging in the types of activities associated with sustaining an independent living situation (eg, shopping, medical appointments, outdoor exercise), they can also interfere with older adults' ability to visit the places many associate with a high quality of life (eg, green spaces, houses of worship, senior centers, the homes of family and friends). Other barriers that may be more common to suburban and rural environments, such as the absence of sidewalks and other walkways, adequate lighting, and public transportation; geographic features such as steep inclines; or natural features such as mud and brush, can render older adults homebound.

House Exterior

On opening their front doors, many older adults are stuck at the top of their own front steps because of broken stairs, a lack of adequate railings, or stairs that are too steep or slippery for increasingly weak leg muscles to navigate. Each time they descend or ascend these steps, these individuals face the risk of falling, which can lead to serious injury or even death. Unsafe stairs pose a threat when older adults must go out (for example, to attend a medical appointment) and also bar exiting the home for optional activities such as volunteer work, socializing with friends and family, or participating in religious services. These disparities in housing conditions can lead to health disparities because community-dwelling older adults derive benefits from social engagement outside their homes, such as caregiving for friends or neighbors,[11,12] working part time,[13] or attending church and family activities.[14] Onset of functional decline, which can put older adults at risk when entering or exiting their homes if proper safety measures are not in place, has been linked to cessation of these types of potentially beneficial activities.[15]

UNSAFE HOME INTERIORS CAN POSE EVEN GREATER THREATS TO AGING WITH INDEPENDENCE

Although unsafe exterior environments, such as communities with neighborhood violence and broken sidewalks, pose some of the most visibly obvious threats to the health and well-being of older persons, often the most dangerous place for these adults is inside their own homes. Interactions between underlying health conditions and unsafe home interiors result in functional limitations that not only place older adults at risk for injury but also prevent them from doing the things they associate with living well. Given the severe challenges of addressing the problems that may exist outside an older adult's home, the rest of this article focuses on strategies for supporting aging with independence by addressing the safety issues that often exist inside older adults' homes and that contribute to functional limitations in later life.

Fall Risk and the Home Environment

One in 3 adults fall every year with subsequent morbidity including nursing home admission and mortality.[16,17] Not only are the falls dangerous but so is remaining on the ground if unable to arise. Individual (intrinsic) factors contributing to falls include decreased mobility, decreased balance, decreased vision, and medications that act on the central nervous system. External (extrinsic) factors are equally important and include clutter, uneven or hole-ridden floors, inadequate railing or banisters, steep stairs, oxygen tubing, wires in walking spaces, and slick surfaces such as bathroom floors. In addition, there are extrinsic factors that are made more dangerous by interactions with intrinsic factors; for example, slippery bathtubs with high sides in the home of someone with poor balance, or toilets without grab bars in the home of someone with weak legs (**Fig. 1**).

Activities of Daily Living/Instrumental Activities of Daily Living and Environmental Factors

Activities of daily living (ADLs), including bathing, grooming, getting on and off of the toilet, getting in and out of the bed, and dressing are, by definition, essential to daily

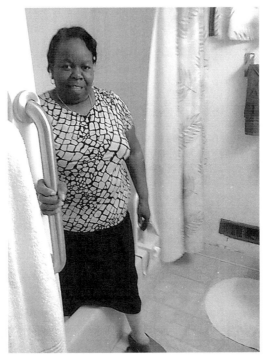

Fig. 1. A client practices using grab bars to exit the bathtub.

life. Community-dwelling older adults who cannot safely do these activities on their own must rely on informal or paid caregivers in order to age in place. Because of a tendency to focus on illness management rather than function, medical and nursing professionals may fail to adequately assess and address older adults' functional challenges, even though function is the key to staying independent. An estimated $350 billion each year are spent on nursing home care for people unable to function independently. An additional $450 billion in unpaid care are provided by informal or family caregivers assisting older adults in performing everyday self-care tasks.[18] Without intervention, these costs will continue to increase as the population ages.

AN INNOVATIVE MODEL FOR PROMOTING AGING WITH INDEPENDENCE: THE CAPABLE INTERVENTION

Practical realities related to both older adults' preferences for living independently and increased demands on families and other caregivers associated with a growing aging population show a clear need to find sustainable models of care that address both the intrinsic and extrinsic factors that improve safety and function in older adults seeking to age in place. First-hand experiences providing house calls to low-income urban community-dwelling older adults brought this need to the forefront of the first author's (Dr Sarah Szanton) attention. Acting in response to the many older adults she had encountered who were struggling to age independently and safely, she found a program called ABLE (Advancing Better Living for Elders) that had already been proved effective in addressing similar challenges. ABLE had previously been evaluated through a randomized controlled trial of 306 older adults in Philadelphia. The program provided occupational and physical therapy sessions involving home modifications and training in their use; instruction in problem-solving strategies, energy conservation, safe performance of ADLS/instrumental ADLs (IADLs) and fall recovery techniques, as well as muscle and balance training. The evaluation of this model provided strong evidence that a program focused on improving community-dwelling older adults' function and control over their circumstances could help to promote aging with independence in these populations and even delay mortality.[19,20] Dr Szanton sought to build on the strengths of ABLE, and also to modify the intervention to address additional threats to aging with independence (such as perilous home environments and their interactions with underlying health issues) more explicitly. The result of these efforts was the CAPABLE intervention. CAPABLE augmented ABLE by adding support for repairs to unsafe home environments (as opposed to strictly home modifications such as grab bars and raised toilet seats) and a nurse who comprehensively assesses and addresses health concerns that could contribute to functional limitations within the home environment, such as pain, depression, medication reconciliation, and primary care provider (PCP) advocacy/communication. These realms were added in the service of increasing clients' capacity to perform ADLs and IADLs independently. The CAPABLE intervention involves universal assessment of every client by a registered nurse (RN)/occupational therapist (OT) team that then allows an interdisciplinary team including the client, the nurse, the OT, a home repair specialist (handyman), and a pharmacist to tailor an individualized plan of care that addresses potential threats to aging independence in the home environment while working toward functional goals set by the client. **Table 1** provides a description of the visits and their sequencing and the protocol and description of what the nurse does in CAPABLE is given by Pho and colleagues.[21]

Between 2009 and 2010, a randomized controlled pilot trial of CAPABLE was conducted with a sample of 40 low-income older adults, randomly assigned to receive the

Table 1
Home visits and collaboration with CAPABLE clients over a 4-month period

Team Member	OT Visit 1[a]	OT Visit 2	After Visit 2	Visit 3	Visit 4	Visit 5	Visit 6
OT and client together	Introduction Function-focused OT assessment. Fall risk and recovery education	Determine client's functional goals, conduct home safety assessment and identify necessary repairs or modifications	Develop work order for home repairs/modifications and sends to HM	Brainstorm and develop action plan with client for client-identified goal #1	Brainstorm and develop action plan with client for client-identified goal #2	Brainstorm and develop action plan with client for identified goal #3 Review HM work and train participant on new assistive devices	Wrap up, help participant generalize solutions for future problems Review goals and client's achievement of them
HM	HM visits client's home, reviews repairs/modifications and associated costs with OT, starts work and continues until complete						

Team Member			RN Visit 1	After RN Visit 1	RN Visit 2	RN Visit 3	RN Visit 4
RN and client together			Introduction Function-focused RN assessment including pain, mood, strength, balance, medication information, health care provider (PCP) advocacy/communication	Make medication calendar for client Review client's medications, including side effects, interactions, and possible changes Consult with pharmacist if on high alert or more than 15 medications	Determine goals in RN domain together, start to brainstorm goals Demonstrate CAPABLE exercises Review, clarify, and modify medication calendar Consider how to improve communication with PCP Develop correspondence to PCP	Complete brainstorming/problem-solving process. Develop action plans with client. Assess PCP response to communication of client needs. Review/assess/troubleshoot exercise regimen	Review progress and use of strategies for all target areas. Complete action plans. Review RN section of flipbook that summarizes program. Evaluate achievement of goals and readiness to change scale

Abbreviation: HM, handyman.

[a] The visits are staggered so that OT visits 1 and 2 occur before RN visit 1. RN only has 4 visits, whereas the OT has 6.

CAPABLE intervention. This pilot showed that those receiving CAPABLE improved on all primary outcomes, compared with a control group, and also had less difficulty with ADLs and IADLs, less pain, and improved falls efficacy.[22] Based on those findings, the CAPABLE team was funded by the National Institutes of Health to conduct a 300-person randomized clinical trial assessing whether the intervention improves function, well-being, and health care costs on a larger scale. Also, the Center for Medicare and Medicaid Innovations, created by the Affordable Care Act, funded the team to provide the CAPABLE intervention to 500 people and test whether the program delayed nursing home admission and preventable hospital costs. Results from these trials will be available between 2015 and 2017. In the meantime, much has been learned about implementing such a program in the community and assessing what is working so far.

THREE INNOVATIONS OF THE CAPABLE MODEL IN ACTION: A CASE EXAMPLE

CAPABLE is innovative in 3 ways. First, it is not just client centered but client directed. Second, unlike most forms of home health care, the nurse and OT strive to address the functional goals of the client, not just their medical issues. Third, the CAPABLE model treats the home environment as a key influence on health, such that fixing up an older adults' home interior is done for the primary purpose of achieving health-related goals. The following case is an example of this 3-pronged CAPABLE approach:

The Client

When first enrolled in CAPABLE, Mrs R was a frail obese woman in her late 60s who experienced debilitating pain and depressive symptoms, had difficulty managing her multiple medications, and lived in an unsafe home environment that put her at risk for falls. Although she described herself as a "people person," functional limitations had limited her ability to go out for activities such as shopping, church, and family gatherings. As a result of lower extremity weakness, holes in her living room floors, kitchen flooring that was sticking up, and lack of environmental supports (railings and other home fixtures), she also had extreme difficulty doing things in her own home. She found difficulty in cooking for herself, going down to her basement, or going up to her second floor.

The Client's Functional Goals

Mrs R expressed a desire to do more in her home, including cooking and improving her ability to access different levels of her house. She wanted to be able to leave the house for activities such as family events and church.

Issues Affecting Goal Achievement and Resulting Interventions

Assessment by the CAPABLE nurse/OT team revealed the following issues affecting Mrs R's safety and ability to achieve her functional goals: medication side effects, symptoms such as pain and low mood, lower extremity weakness, and unsafe walkways and stairways in the home. Working collaboratively with other members of the interdisciplinary team over a 4-month period, the CAPABLE nurse worked to address these issues in a manner tailored to Mrs R's unique circumstances and home environment.

Medication side effects

When she enrolled in CAPABLE, Mrs R took both Celebrex 200 mg twice a day and Motrin 200 to 400 mg 4 times a day as needed for pain. In addition, Mrs R had 3 to 4+ edema in her lower extremities. On noting the edema, the CAPABLE nurse reached out to Mrs R's PCP to suggest discontinuing the Celebrex. The nurse then suggested replacing the nonsteroidal antiinflammatory drugs with Tylenol, Voltaren topical cream, and exercise.

Pain and low mood

Mrs R's depressive symptoms, in combination with her pain, were a barrier to many types of activity including standing long enough to cook for herself and socializing with others. Following the nursing intervention regarding her prescription to Celebrex, Mrs R started Tylenol instead. She continued to take Motrin on occasion. Mrs R stated that since her pain had decreased, her mood had improved. She began cooking for herself and her family, and began making trial runs to family gatherings, building toward her ultimate goal of attending church services.

Lower extremity weakness

Lack of strength in her lower extremities prevented Mrs R from walking around as well as leaving her home. The RN taught Mrs R a series of simple lower extremity exercises. On the first nursing visit, Mrs R had so much difficulty demonstrating the exercises she had been taught (because of pain) that the CAPABLE nurse thought Mrs R would not continue exercising on her own. However, the adjustments to Mrs R's medications, in addition to the exercise, started to make a difference. Mrs R began exercising more regularly and asked the nurse for more advanced exercises on subsequent visits. She also started a walking routine inside the house after the handyman had fixed the holes in her floors and the kitchen linoleum trip hazard.

Lack of railings on stairways

The lack of second railings on stairs to the basement and upper floor of the house constituted a serious fall risk for Mrs R that impeded her from navigating her own home. The CAPABLE handyman installed second railings on both the stairs to the second floor and to the basement. Mrs R reported that the second railing had made going up and down the steps much easier and safer. She said, "You all have made my life easier. I was going up the steps on my hands and knees and coming down the steps sideways. I now have the 2 banisters where I can come down safely, facing forward holding onto both banisters."

Value Added by the CAPABLE Approach

An older adult with Mrs R's risk profile is likely to have been admitted to a hospital or a nursing home over time, because of her multimorbidities, multiple medications, social isolation, and frail physical and emotional state.[23] The CAPABLE team took an innovative approach to addressing these challenges by focusing on Mrs R's functional goals, rather than solely addressing medical issues. Taking their cues from Mrs R, an interprofessional team consisting of a nurse, an OT, a pharmacist, and a handyman designed a 3-pronged combination of functional, medical, and environmental adjustments that worked synergistically over a 4-month period to meet Mrs R's unique needs within her home environment.

Innovation 1: client-directed care

Mrs R's goals became the CAPABLE team's goals and directed development of the plan of care. The team's efforts to improve pain control, medication management, and strength/balance were in the service of Mrs R's overall goals to cook for herself, get around and out of the house, and eventually to attend church services.

Innovation 2: addressing medical/functional issues through an RN/OT team

In a similar way, nursing assessment and related interventions were driven by functional (rather than strictly medical) goals of the client and were designed to complement

Table 2
Role differences between the traditional home health RN and the CAPABLE RN

Role	Home Health RN	CAPABLE RN
Goal-setting and plan of care	Nurse-driven goal-setting and plan of care centered on the patient illness or injury as identified by the client's health care provider	Client-driven goal-setting and plan of care centered on the functional goals and activities of interest identified by the client
Collaboration with client	RN works as a treatment provider to the client for a specific medical problem as directed by the client's health care provider RN-delivered treatments based on prescriptions from client's health care provider	RN serves as a consultant to clients for achieving their functional goals In partnership with the client, the RN helps to determine and shape the intervention by paying special attention to the clients' preferences, pain, mood, medications, fall risk, and strength/balance
Interdisciplinary collaborations	RN works apart from other specialists, but refers client to specialists and other services as needed (eg, physical or occupational therapy, social work)	RN works as an integral part of an interdisciplinary team that includes the client, an OT, a home improvement specialist, and a pharmacist. RN refers client to social work services from local agencies as needed
Provision of skilled nursing care	Skilled nursing care (eg, physical assessment, phlebotomy, administration of intravenous medications, wound care, patient education) provided as prescribed by client's health care provider	Skilled nursing care provided as needed to meet client-directed functional goals of care, in consultation with interdisciplinary team Client's health care provider alerted to medical situations and to recommend adjustments to medications/therapies requiring a prescription Examples: orthostatic hypotension, foot wounds

Focus on medications	RN reconciles client's medications with a general focus on side effects. Notifies client's health care provider of significant interactions. Client education provided as needed	RN reconciles client's medications with a specific focus on falls prevention and high-alert medications. Notifies client's health care provider of significant interactions. Additional activities include: • Creates medication calendar for client • Assesses for and advises client on issues related to medication adherence • Assesses medications with focus on reducing client costs • Works with pharmacist in situations in which client is on high-alert medications or more than 15 medications
Focus on pain	RN performs general assessment for pain and more specific assessments as directed by client's illness or injury. Client education provided as needed	At each visit, RN performs thorough assessment for pain with a focus on how pain affects client function and progress toward client-identified goals of care Based on assessment, RN provides client-specific education on pain identification, alleviation, or prevention, and pharmacologic and nonpharmacologic approaches to pain management
Duration of care	Home health services provided for up to 60 d per episode of care as defined by Medicare; RN visit frequency may vary	CAPABLE intervention delivered over 4 mo; RN sees client a maximum of 4 visits
Other demands on RN	RN may supervise other home health workers (licensed practical nurses or home health aides) RN may be on-call nights, weekends, or holidays RN may regularly do extensive bending, lifting, or standing	RN does not supervise other home health workers No need for RN coverage on nights, weekends, or holidays Limited amount of bending/lifting (required only on occasion)

Table 3
Recommendations to nurses collaborating with OTs

Recommendation	Application to CAPABLE Study	Specific Example
Understand the OT's scope of practice	When working with CAPABLE clients, nurses recognize the OT's role in promoting client independence and function by: • Promoting clients' own strategies to maintain and improve different areas of their lives amplified with OT clinical knowledge • Facilitating client's access to and use of durable medical equipment and adaptive equipment, as appropriate • Prioritizing necessary modifications to client's home environment	A client goal is fall prevention. In a typical CAPABLE plan of care, the OT brainstorms with the client safe ways to get into the bath and training on using new grab bars and railings inside or outside the house, and so forth. The nurse complements but does not duplicate the OT role by focusing on client's medications, nutrition, and disease and symptom management, all of which can also lead to falls
Maintain constant communication with the OT and other interdisciplinary team members	As in any other health care environment, open communication leads to better client outcomes and success Determine the personality and communication styles within the team and use appropriate communication strategies, as needed	The nurse attends routine meetings of the interdisciplinary team and maintains regular communication with OTs (via phone, email, or face to face) to debrief following client visits and to discuss collaborative approaches to meeting emerging client needs and strengths
Be aware of OT's activities with clients and reinforce when appropriate	By maintaining excellent communication and familiarizing themselves with client goals and the plan of care (including activities of each of the interdisciplinary team members), nurses reinforce OT activities/teaching when interacting with CAPABLE clients	The nurse teaches balance and strength exercises. The OT works with a client to use assistive devices such as walkers or home modifications such as railings and grab bars. The OT reminds the client to perform the exercises. On subsequent visits, the nurse watches the clients use appropriate assistive devices/home modifications

and reinforce the activities of an OT. Working as an RN/OT team, in conjunction with other specialists such as the handyman and the pharmacist, the two types of clinicians were able to implement a plan of care that helped Mrs R to meet her functional goals.

Innovation 3: treating housing as health

The efforts of the RN/OT team would not have been as successful without the addition of important safety measures within Mrs R's home environment. Mrs R had many small alterations to her home that helped her function there independently as well as to get out to her important activities. In turn, these should help her health costs through increased activities and quality of life.

Through these efforts, the CAPABLE team sought to reverse the vicious cycle that affects so many older adults with similar risk profiles as Mrs R, who become increasingly deconditioned, depressed, and frail over time. The hope is that consequently these actions will also decrease Mrs R's future risk for serious medical consequences, injury, or further functional declines that would require costly care.[23]

LESSONS LEARNED WHILE IMPLEMENTING THE CAPABLE MODEL

To date, implementation of the prior pilot randomized controlled trial and larger on-going clinical trials funded by the National Institutes of Health and the Centers for Medicare and Medicaid Services- has taught the CAPABLE research team valuable lessons about improving unsafe home environments and supporting aging independence by applying a client-directed model of care, addressing both medical and functional issues using an interdisciplinary team approach, and incorporating home repair into health care.

1. Lessons learned about client-directed care. In our experience, prioritizing the clients' goals makes clients likely to follow through. When clients say they are worried about falls, and the CAPABLE nurse presents core strengthening exercises to help prevent falls, then the client is likely to follow through on the exercises because they relate to the goal. Client-directed care can be hard at first for the RN to get used to because RNs are used to having medical goals and imparting them to the client. See **Table 2** for lessons learned about how the CAPABLE RN role is different from home care RN.
2. Lessons learned about addressing medical and functional issues through an interdisciplinary team. Similar to addressing the client's goals, addressing the specific functional goals is the key to motivation. Clients are often not as concerned about their medical disease as they are about the ability to function. When both are addressed, it is a support for the client to be able to live with independence and dignity and leads to durable uptake of the new strategies. See **Table 3** for recommendations to nurses collaborating with OTs.
3. Lessons learned about housing/environment as health. The changes to the home environment are durable and serve as visible reminders for clients to approach their daily functions with their new CAPABLE approaches. After CAPABLE is over, if someone forgets to take their pain medications, they will still have repaired holes, taped down rugs, and sturdy banisters to help them move around the home with increased function. It is hoped that these extrinsic changes will work with the intrinsic changes and new problem-solving strategies to approach inevitable new issues as they age.

SUMMARY

Aging with independence is important for older adults. Independence means not only living in one's home but also being able to choose how to spend one's days. Both of these rely on function, which is a product of the interaction of health and the environment. Drawing on successful interventions and clinical experience, we developed an innovative program that (1) allows clients to set their own goals; (2) involves an interdisciplinary team addressing issues of function and medical problems to help clients meet their goals; (3) treats the housing and the environment as an aspect of health care worthy of health care investment. This article shares the lessons learned in the project. If current testing is successful according to the actuaries at the Centers for Medicare and Medicaid Services, CAPABLE can be scaled up nationally through the Affordable Care Act. If this happens, the lessons learned and the resources we have developed will be important to explore in different contexts and states. It is hoped that this program, designed to improve lives and independence, will also save health care costs for families and the nation.

REFERENCES

1. Schwanen T, Ziegler F. Wellbeing, independence, and mobility: an introduction. Ageing Soc 2011;31(5):719–33.
2. US Census Bureau. American community survey, 2007-2011, detailed tables. 2013. Available at: www.socialexplorer.com/home. Accessed June 2, 2013.
3. Green CR, Anderson KO, Baker TA, et al. The unequal burden of pain: confronting racial and ethnic disparities in pain. Pain Med 2003;4(3):277–94.
4. Minkler M, Fuller-Thomson E, Guralnik JM. Gradient of disability across the socioeconomic spectrum in the United States. N Engl J Med 2006;355(7):695–703.
5. Fuller-Thomson E, Nuru-Jeter A, Minkler M, et al. Black-white disparities in disability among older Americans: further untangling the role of race and socioeconomic status. J Aging Health 2009;21(5):677–98.
6. Szanton SL, Gill JM. Facilitating resilience using a society-to-cells framework: a theory of nursing essentials applied to research and practice. ANS Adv Nurs Sci 2010;33(4):329–43.
7. Roman CG, Chalfin A. Fear of walking outdoors. A multilevel ecologic analysis of crime and disorder. Am J Prev Med 2008;34(4):306–12.
8. Rauh VA, Landrigan PJ, Claudio L. Housing and health: intersection of poverty and environmental exposures. Ann N Y Acad Sci 2008;1136:276–88.
9. Aneshensel CS, Wight RG, Miller-Martinez D, et al. Urban neighborhoods and depressive symptoms among older adults. J Gerontol B Psychol Sci Soc Sci 2007;62(1):S52–9.
10. Warren-Findlow J. Weathering: stress and heart disease in African American women living in Chicago. Qual Health Res 2006;16(2):221–37.
11. Martinez IL, Crooks D, Kim KS, et al. Invisible civic engagement among older adults: valuing the contributions of informal volunteering. J Cross Cult Gerontol 2011;26(1):23–37.
12. Hinterlong JE. Productive engagement among older Americans: prevalence, patterns, and implications for public policy. J Aging Soc Policy 2008;20(2):141–64.
13. Kampfe CM, Wadsworth JS, Mamboleo GI, et al. Aging, disability, and employment. Work 2008;31(3):337–44.
14. Hybels CF, Blazer DG, George LK, et al. The complex association between religious activities and functional limitations in older adults. Gerontologist 2012;52(5):676–85.
15. Butrica BA, Johnson RW, Zedlewski SR. Volunteer dynamics of older Americans. J Gerontol B Psychol Sci Soc Sci 2009;64(5):644–55.
16. Hu G, Baker SP. Recent increases in fatal and non-fatal injury among people aged 65 years and over in the USA. Inj Prev 2010;16:26–30.

17. Gill TM, Murphy TE, Gahbauer EA, et al. Association of injurious falls with disability outcomes and nursing home admissions in community-living older persons. Am J Epidemiol 2013;178(3):418–25.

18. Feinberg L, Reinhard SC. Valuing the invaluable: 2011 update. The growing contributions and costs of family caregiving. Washington, DC: AARP Public Policy institute; 2011.

19. Gitlin LN, Hauck WW, Dennis MP, et al. Long-term effect on mortality of a home intervention that reduces functional difficulties in older adults: results from a randomized trial. J Am Geriatr Soc 2009;57(3):476–81.

20. Gitlin LN, Winter L, Dennis MP, et al. A randomized trial of a multicomponent home intervention to reduce functional difficulties in older adults. J Am Geriatr Soc 2006;54(5):809–16.

21. Pho AT, Tanner EK, Roth J, et al. Nursing strategies for promoting and maintaining function among community-living older adults: the CAPABLE intervention. Geriatr Nurs 2012;33(6):439–45.

22. Szanton SL, Thorpe RJ, Boyd C, et al. Community aging in place, advancing better living for elders: a bio-behavioral-environmental intervention to improve function and health-related quality of life in disabled older adults. J Am Geriatr Soc 2011;59(12):2314–20.

23. Woods NF, LaCroix AZ, Gray SL, et al. Frailty: emergence and consequences in women aged 65 and older in the women's health initiative observational study. J Am Geriatr Soc 2005;53(8):1321–30.

Maintenance of Physical Function in Frail Older Adults

Carol E. Rogers, PhD, RN[a],*, Maria Cordeiro, MS, APRN, CNP[b], Erica Perryman, BBA[c]

KEYWORDS

- Physical activity • Sedentary • Community • Low intensity • Frailty
- Physical function

KEY POINTS

- Participating in regular physical activity is safe for sedentary older adults.
- Multiple barriers prevent the initiation and maintenance of a regular routine of physical activity.
- Health care provider recommendations are important to changing behavior.
- Social settings, such as a faith-based community, may be the social–relational connection or key ingredient of the intervention delivery.

Physical function tends to decrease with older Americans, while disability rates usually increase with age.[1] These changes may impair mobility and functional capacity that ultimately affect quality of life and lead to institutionalization. Although much of the general public mistakenly believes this decline is inevitable, loss of function is not a part of normal aging. One key factor in the prevention of functional decline is participation in regular physical activity (PA). Older adults are still capable of caring for themselves, and some continue to compete as elite athletes into their 90s (eg, Jack LaLanne, who became a TV fitness icon for women from 1952 to 1985, and continued

Funding sources: Dr C.E. Rogers, E. Perryman: None; M. Cordeiro: Reynolds Center of Geriatric Nursing Excellence Scholarship.
Conflict of Interest: None.
[a] Department of Nursing, Donald W Reynolds Center of Geriatric Nursing Excellence, College of Nursing, University of Oklahoma Health Sciences Center, 1100 North Stonewall Avenue, Office 410, Oklahoma City, OK 73120, USA; [b] Department of Nursing, Reynolds Center of Geriatric Nursing Excellence, College of Nursing, University of Oklahoma Health Sciences Center, 1300 Olde North Place, Edmond, OK 73034, USA; [c] Department of Nursing, Reynolds Center of Geriatric Nursing Excellence, College of Nursing, University of Oklahoma Health Sciences Center, 1100 North Stonewall Avenue, Office 472, Oklahoma City, OK 73117, USA
* Corresponding author.
E-mail address: Carol-rogers@ouhsc.edu

his daily 2-hour workout as a nonagenarian).[2] More importantly, women enjoyed working out with Jack. His workouts were easily performed in the home with low-cost, low-tech equipment.

Despite the popularity of numerous televised exercise programs and more than a decade of national attempts to increase participation in regular PA, older adults in the United States are sedentary. Only 20% participate in strength training required to maintain physical function.[2] As older adults transition to retirement, many lose the benefits gained from occupational or lifestyle PA.[3] To make a significant impact on this national trend, it is critical that health care providers actively screen older adults to determine if they are meeting the national requirements for PA and provide recommendations for sedentary older adults. Research evidence shows that low-intensity physical activity is feasible and beneficial for older adults.[4] This article will review strategies to reduce the barriers and strengthen motivators to this important behavior change for frail older adults. Research continues to develop and test strategies to support frail older adults who need to initiate and maintain a regular routine of PA.

BACKGROUND

Older adults generally fall into 5 categories of physical functionality that range from physically elite to physically independent.[5] Physically elite older adults are master athletes who train on a daily basis or continue to work in a physically demanding profession such as a hiking instructor or firefighter. Physically fit older adults remain very active, exercising intentionally 2 to 7 days a week, and may continue working. Physically independent older adults do not exercise with any regularity, but have not been diagnosed with a debilitating disease known to result in loss of function and independence. These older adults have little physical reserve and are close to transitioning to the next level of function, which is physically frail.

Physically frail older adults are able to perform activities of daily living that are basic to caring for oneself.[5] They may require some assistance such as meal preparation and shopping to maintain independence. Frailty is not the same as disability, but frail older adults are at risk of developing a disability and death from a minor stressor.[5] Frailty is a geriatric syndrome that results from impaired physiologic reserve across multiple systems.[6] That loss of reserve may be due to age, disease, or disuse. It results in a reduced ability to withstand physical and psychosocial stressors and increases an older person's vulnerability to adverse mental and physical health outcomes.[6] Clinical symptoms may include anorexia, weight loss, fatigue, and inactivity; signs include reduced immune function, age-related muscle wasting (sarcopenia), age-related loss of muscle strength (dynapenia), bone thinning (osteopenia), malnutrition, balance disturbance, and gait instability. Key factors leading to the development of frailty are chronic undernutrition and physical inactivity.[6] Predictably, the outcomes associated with frailty are increased risk of falls with injury, acute illness, cognitive decline, disability, dependency, social isolation, institutionalization, and death.[6] Clearly, it is important to be proactive in the management and prevention of frailty in older adults, because the associated functional decline is costly to the individual; additionally, the associated higher health care resource utilization is costly to the larger society.

The lowest level of physical function is physically dependent, which is characterized as inability to complete some or all of the activities of daily living and depend upon others for basic needs. When the demands of self-care outweigh the homeostatic reserves of the older adult, the frail elder is no longer able to independently meet day-to-day functional needs and becomes dependent on formal or informal assistance; this, potentially, leads to institutionalization.[5,6] Disability rates are higher in centenarians and tend to be higher in women, African Americans, and those below the federal poverty levels.[1]

MANAGEMENT

Management of frailty begins with the identification and management of underlying disease states that are associated with anorexia and wasting disorders. These states include medical conditions such as congestive heart failure or diabetes as well as psychological conditions such as depression or dementia. Once underlying chronic conditions are addressed, management of frailty must focus on such supportive and preventive interventions as a regular routine of physical activity to improve or maintain physical function. The health benefits of physical activity contribute to reducing risk of the progression to frailty and extend beyond physical function. In particular, the evidence is clear that engaging in a routine of regular exercise is helpful in 2 areas. It not only builds strength, flexibility, balance, and endurance, but it also protects against, and helps manage, chronic conditions such as cardiovascular disease, diabetes, cancer, and osteoporosis,[7] in older adults.[8,9] Both pathways ultimately contribute to improved physical function in older adults.

EVALUATION/DIAGNOSIS

Two annual screening activities that may identify the risk for progression of functional decline toward physical dependence are the amount of physical activity in which an older adult participates on a regular basis and his or her functional fitness levels. These screens compliment the annual review of health systems and chronic conditions. A decline in activity from 1 year to the next is an indicator that an older adult needs a prescription for PA to maintain his or her ability to perform the activities of daily living required to maintain independence. When asked about level of activity, most will give the answer they think the questioner desires. For example, patients may say with confidence they walk every day, but simply observing the pace of walking into the office informs the assessment negatively. Questions asking for simple yes or no responses usually do not provide enough information. Barriers to using more complex screening tools include the time involved. Multiple screening surveys for PA are available, but many require over 15 minutes to administer and even more time to score. The Stanford Brief Physical Activity Survey offers the least burden on the patient and health care provider; it takes less than 5 minutes to administer and score according to level of physical activity.[10] The tool takes into account the typical activities over the course of a year and includes lifestyle activities such as yard work and household cleaning. Based on the level of physical activity, health care providers can make the needed recommendations for PA.

Functional fitness components required to perform the activities of daily living required for the maintenance of independence include cardiorespiratory fitness, musculoskeletal fitness, balance, flexibility, motor agility, and body composition.[5,11] Rikli and Jones developed a battery of tests to assess these areas of functional fitness[12] that are easy to administer and require minimal equipment and space. Normal scores have been scaled according to age and gender, allowing for interpretation of the initial findings. The scores also provide an objective measure to monitor changes in fitness over the course of time. Health care providers can also tailor a prescription for PA based on the findings of the screen. For example, if an individual scores in the 50th percentile for the flexibility measures, but in the 25th percentile for strength measures, an appropriate exercise would include strength training. The logical next step is to make recommendations for initiating a regular routine and follow-up of PA.

RECOMMENDATIONS FOR PA

The goal of promoting PA in physically independent and frail older adults is to prevent the decline to physical dependence. The American Heart Association and American College of Sports Medicine national physical activity guidelines for older adults recommend moderate-intensity aerobic activity for a minimum of 30 minutes 5 days a week or vigorous aerobic activity 20 minutes 3 days a week.[4] In addition, patients should participate in strength training and endurance exercises 2 days per week, with balance and flexibility exercises 2 days per week for 10 minutes.[4] Assurance to the individual should include the message that it is never too late to start a exercising. Frail and deconditioned older adults must start slow with a routine of strength, balance, and flexibility training to build endurance prior to participating in moderate-intensity physical activity.[4] There is evidence that some health benefits are achieved with as little as 2 exercise sessions per week.[13]

Older adults are more likely to engage in a regular routine of PA when their health care provider gives them a recommendation to do so.[13] That recommendation is more effective when it is in writing, just like a prescription for a medication. Prescriptions are more effective when they include the type, frequency, and specific duration of PA sessions.[4,14,15] The prescription also needs to account for the older adults specific needs. For example, an older adult with poor balance may need to start with some balance training prior to initiating a walking intervention, whether it is indoors or outdoors. Older adults are more likely to change their behavior if the health care provider explores the patients' expectations of initiating a new routine of PA[16] and feel in control.[17] Some older adults may require monitored sessions to build endurance prior to exercising independently. Due to the uncertainty of health care providers to give the appropriate recommendation, many older adults do not receive any information, remain sedentary, and lose the ability to care for themselves. The Exercise Assessment and Screening for You (EASY) tool is available online[18] at http://www.easyforyou.info/ and in print to help older adults and health care providers select activities that are safe and effective based on individual responses to a set of 6 questions.[19] Questions refer to the individual's experiencing chest pains or pressure on exertion, dizziness or feeling lightheaded, high blood pressure, unsteadiness, pain or physical symptoms preventing PA, or other reasons a patient might be concerned about starting a PA program.[18] Use of this tool has enabled older adults with major health problems to enroll in and successfully complete fall prevention classes.[20]

PATIENT CONSIDERATIONS TO INITIATING AND MAINTAINING A ROUTINE OF PA

Multiple considerations are necessary in initiating and maintaining a routine of PA for older adults. Health care providers may need to help older adults remove barriers and recognize facilitators to making this important health behavior change.

Barriers

Multiple barriers to initiating and maintaining a regular routine of physical activity are reported in the literature specific to older adults.[11,14,21] Cultural and geographic populations studied include African American,[22–26] Australian,[27] Canadian,[28] Russian immigrant,[29] Asian,[30] Korean,[31] German,[32] Latino,[25,33,34] Italian,[35] Swedish,[36] Norwegian,[37] Chinese,[25] Vietnamese,[25] American Indian,[25] Israeli,[38] and multiethnic populations.[39] Health-related populations studied have included persons with obesity,[17,26] arthritis,[40] Alzheimer disease (and caregivers),[41] diabetes,[24] Parkinson disease,[42] cardiovascular disease,[43,44] sleep,[16] cancer,[45,46] mobility disabilities,[26] depression,[47] and multiple sclerosis.[48] It has been found that some barriers are consistent for older adults across many cultures and diagnoses.

The environmental barriers of safety include uneven sidewalks, lack of streetlights, high crime rates, extreme temperatures, dangerous crosswalks, lack of facilities in community, and high cost of the program.[11,14,49] Uneven sidewalks is one of the top risk of falls in older adults who may walk with a shuffled gait or do not see the sidewalk due to vision problems or poor lighting. Lack of streetlights decreases visibility while walking early in the morning or later in the evening, which may be necessary to avoid exposure and exertion in the heat of summer or accommodate for work schedules. Lack of streetlights is also associated with higher crime rates. Extreme temperatures are of particular concern in communities that are extremely hot in the summer or cold in the winter.[50] Many busy intersections lack stoplights to allow safe crossing. The timing of crosswalk traffic is often not long enough to allow persons with slow gait speed to cross before allowing the flow of traffic to proceed. Additional barriers include communities with lack of facilities with PA programs and equipment, no transportation to facilities, and high program costs.[11,21]

Intrapersonal barriers to initiating PA for frail older adults are numerous and include beliefs about negative effects of PA, physically inability to perform a PA activity, lack of confidence in ability to exercise, no time to exercise, fatigue, concern for appearance, and previous negative experience with PA. Negative beliefs about PA include fears that it will increase arthritis pain[40] or a fall, that patients are too ill for PA,[21,35,51] or that PA might worsen conditions following a unilateral stroke.[44] Physical limitations cited by individuals that keep them from participating in regular PA include shortness of breath and leg problems,[52] fatigue from caregiving of others with Alzheimer disease,[41] or diabetes-related comorbid conditions.[53]

Lack of time is a common barrier to exercise. One planning strategy is to ask patients what time of the day would be best for adding a new activity to their already busy schedule. African American and Latino traditions reflect the precedence of care of family members over self-care activities including PA.[33,34,41,43,50] Family caregivers in general may state similar beliefs. One way to help overcome this barrier is to actually involve the family in the planned activity or include family members in the discussion about ways for the caregiver to arrange time. A theme unique to frail older adults is that many feel they are too old to change their activity.[36] This can be more easily overcome by providing specific examples of ways to initiate change slowly and safely as demonstrated by other older adults like themselves.

Walking is an outstanding exemple of a low-cost, low-intensity PA for older adults. The most common barrier is the outdoors environment. It is often too hot or cold for frail older adults to walk outdoors.[51] Before recommending outside walking for frail older adults, assess a safe walking path and time whether busy intersections have stoplights that are active long enough to cross safely. Some communities have built outdoor walking tracks to increase walking for PA in all generations. Some shopping malls encourage walking and provide covered protection for older adults, providing distance markers and seating along the walking route. Other ways to avoid outdoor barriers is using a treadmill. However, treadmills are not without barriers, including difficulty for those with gait problems such as slow walking speed or shuffled foot fall patterns. Most treadmills do not start slow enough to accommodate the older adult's slow gait speed.

Facilitators

The involvement of a group or at least a partner in PA is not only a facilitator, but also helpful keeping up adherence to a program or activity. For walking, it also provides a degree of safety in case there is need for assistance during the walk. Facilitators to older adults initiating and maintaining a routine of PA include tangible improvement, social support, and confidence in one's ability to perform the exercise.[54] In particular, persons with Parkinson disease and multiple sclerosis are more likely to initiate and maintain a regular routine of PA when they believe it will improve their health by slowing disease progression or decline in physical function.[42,55] Persons with arthritis are similarly motivated by expectations of decreased joint pain.[54] Other facilitators to initiating a new routine of PA include having an instructor, having content repeated, reassuring instruction, optimism that the PA will improve chronic disease, and classes taught in a safe environment.[54,56] African American women reported that they found prayer a motivating factor.[57] Family support was an important facilitator to keeping a regular routine of PA in 2 studies of African American and Hispanic older adults.[22,50] The prescription for exercise, discussed earlier, warrants mention again. Individuals are more likely to exercise when they know what specific type of exercise is going to provide them the most benefit, how much is enough to start, what outcomes to look for, and where to find safe classes. Some communities offer a various low-cost, safe PA classes at senior centers, churches, and libraries (**Fig. 1**). In areas where they do not exist, community organizations or senior groups are possible sources for programs to start walking activities or low-exertion PA for frail older adults.

Summary of Recommendations

Specific PA must be predicated on the older adults existing limitations and potential for safe, gradual, improvement. The following approaches are recommended for the frail older adult:

- Screen for level of PA annually
- If physically active, encourage to continue with routine and consult if health interferes with ability to engage in regular physical activity
- If walking is possible, develop a list of safe walking routes
- Locate reputable PA classes in the community
- If sedentary:
  - Screen for prefrail or frailty
  - Discuss the importance of PA for patients based upon their needs
  - Discuss patients goals for the future and how PA can help achieve goals
  - Determine what types of PA are enjoyable for the individual

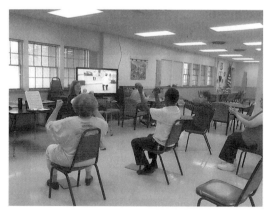

Fig. 1. Example of a physical activity class for older adults.

o Write a prescription for PA with specific dose
o Provide a list of resources in the community

SUMMARY

Annual screening for lifestyle PA and functional changes based on the individual's level of function is critical. The follow-up to screening includes a prescription for PA based on the older adult's needs. The prescription alone is not enough. To reduce the risk of frailty, older adults need to know the type and amount of activity they should engage in plus neighborhood resources for safe, low-cost PA classes taught by individuals who understand the needs of older adults.

REFERENCES

1. National Center for Health Statistics. Health, United States, 2012: with special feature on emergency care. Hyattsville (MD): U.S. Department of Health & Human Services Centers for Disease Control and Prevention; 2013.
2. Wikipedia C. Jack LaLanne. 2013. Available at: http://en.wikipedia.org/wiki/Jack_LaLanne. Accessed October 2, 2013.
3. Slingerland AS, van Lenthe FJ, Jukema JW, et al. Aging, retirement, and changes in physical activity: prospective cohort findings from the GLOBE study. Am J Epidemiol 2007;165(12):1356–63.
4. Nelson ME, Rejeski WJ, Blair SN, et al. Physical activity and public health in older adults: recommendation from the American College of Sports Medicine and the American Heart Association. Med Sci Sports Exerc 2007;39(8):1435–45.
5. Spirduso WW, Francis KL, MacRae PG. Physical dimensions of aging, vol. 2. Champaign (IL): Human Kinetics; 2005.
6. Fried LP, Walston JD, Ferrucci L. Frailty. In: Halter JB, Ouslander JG, Tinetti ME, et al, editors. Hazzard's geriatric medicine and gerontology, vol. 6. New York: McGraw Hill Medical; 2009. p. 632–45.
7. Warburton DE, Nicol CW, Bredin SS. Health benefits of physical activity: the evidence. CMAJ 2006;174(6):801–9.
8. Jahnke R, Larkey L, Rogers CE. Dissemination and benefits of a replicable tai chi and qigong program for older adults. Geriatr Nurs 2010;31(4):272–80.
9. Rogers CE, Larkey LK, Keller C. A review of clinical trials of tai chi and qigong in older adults. West J Nurs Res 2009;31(2):245–79.
10. Taylor-Piliae RE, Fair JM, Haskell WL, et al. Validation of the Stanford brief activity survey: examining psychological factors and physical activity levels in older adults. J Phys Act Health 2010;7(1):87–94.
11. Chodzko-Zajko WJ. ACSM's exercise for older adults. Philadelphia: Wolters Kluwer/Lippincott Williams & Wilkins; 2014.
12. Rikli RE, Jones CJ. Senior fitness test manual. 2nd edition. Champaign (IL): Human Kinetics; 2012.
13. Warburton DE, Nicol CW, Bredin SS. Prescribing exercise as preventive therapy. CMAJ 2006;174(7):961–74.
14. Adams-Fryatt A. Facilitating successful aging: encouraging older adults to be physically active. J Nurse Pract 2010;6(3):187–92.
15. McPhail S, Schippers M. An evolving perspective on physical activity counselling by medical professionals. BMC Fam Pract 2012;13(1):31.
16. Igelstrom H, Martin C, Emtner M, et al. Physical activity in sleep apnea and obesity—personal incentives, challenges, and facilitators for success. Behav Sleep Med 2012;10(2):122–37.

17. Jewson E, Spittle M, Casey M. A preliminary analysis of barriers, intentions, and attitudes towards moderate physical activity in women who are overweight. J Sci Med Sport 2008;11(6):558–61.

18. Texas A&M Health Science Center. EASY: Exercise And Screening for You. Program on Healthy Aging, School of Rural Public Health. 2008. Available at: http://www.easyforyou.info/. Accessed October 2, 2013.

19. Resnick B, Ory MG, Hora K, et al. The Exercise Assessment and Screening for You (EASY) tool: application in the oldest old population. Am J Lifestyle Med 2008;2(5):432–40.

20. Smith ML, Ory MG, Ahn S, et al. Older adults' participation in a community-based falls prevention exercise program: relationships between the EASY tool, program attendance, and health outcomes. Gerontologist 2011;51(6):809–21.

21. Buman MP, Daphna Yasova L, Giacobbi PR. Descriptive and narrative reports of barriers and motivators to physical activity in sedentary older adults. Psychol Sport Exerc 2010;11(3):223–30.

22. Dunn MZ. Psychosocial mediators of a walking intervention among African American women. J Transcult Nurs 2008;19(1):40–6.

23. Hooker SP, Wilcox S, Rheaume CE, et al. Factors related to physical activity and recommended intervention strategies as told by midlife and older African American men. Ethn Dis 2011;21(3):261–7.

24. Komar-Samardzija M, Braun LT, Keithley JK, et al. Factors associated with physical activity levels in African-American women with type 2 diabetes. J Am Acad Nurse Pract 2012;24(4):209–17.

25. Mathews AE, Laditka SB, Laditka JN, et al. Older adults' perceived physical activity enablers and barriers: a multicultural perspective. J Aging Phys Act 2010; 18(2):119.

26. Rimmer JH, Hsieh K, Graham BC, et al. Barrier removal in increasing physical activity levels in obese African American women with disabilities. J Womens Health (Larchmt) 2010;19(10):1869–76.

27. Thomas S, Halbert J, Mackintosh S, et al. Sociodemographic factors associated with self-reported exercise and physical activity behaviors and attitudes of South Australians: results of a population-based survey. J Aging Health 2012; 24(2):287–306.

28. Pan SY, Cameron C, Desmeules M, et al. Individual, social, environmental, and physical environmental correlates with physical activity among Canadians: a cross-sectional study. BMC Public Health 2009;9:21.

29. Purath J, Van Son C, Corbett CF. Physical activity: exploring views of older Russian-speaking Slavic immigrants. Nurs Res Pract 2011;2011:507829.

30. Horne M, Skelton DA, Speed S, et al. Attitudes and beliefs to the uptake and maintenance of physical activity among community-dwelling South Asians aged 60-70 years: a qualitative study. Public Health 2012;126(5):417–23.

31. Park S, Park YH. Predictors of physical activity in Korean older adults: distinction between urban and rural areas. J Korean Acad Nurs 2010;40(2):191–201.

32. Moschny A, Platen P, Klaassen-Mielke R, et al. Barriers to physical activity in older adults in Germany: a cross-sectional study. Int J Behav Nutr Phys Act 2011;8:121.

33. Greaney ML, Lees FD, Lynch B, et al. Using focus groups to identify factors affecting healthful weight maintenance in Latino immigrants. J Nutr Educ Behav 2012;44(5):448–53.

34. Vaughn S. Factors influencing the participation of middle-aged and older Latin American women in physical activity: a stroke-prevention behavior. Rehabil Nurs 2009;34(1):17–23.

35. Bird S, Kurowski W, Feldman S, et al. The influence of the built environment and other factors on the physical activity of older women from different ethnic communities. J Women Aging 2009;21(1):33–47.

36. Leavy B, Aberg AC. "Not ready to throw in the towel": perceptions of physical activity held by older adults in Stockholm and Dublin. J Aging Phys Act 2010; 18(2):219–36.

37. Van Dyck D, De Greef K, Deforche B, et al. Mediators of physical activity change in a behavioral modification program for type 2 diabetes patients. Int J Behav Nutr Phys Act 2011;8:105.

38. Cohen-Mansfield J, Shmotkin D, Goldberg S. Predictors of longitudinal changes in older adults' physical activity engagement. J Aging Phys Act 2010;18(2): 141–57.

39. Mansfield ED, Ducharme N, Koski KG. Individual, social and environmental factors influencing physical activity levels and behaviours of multiethnic socio-economically disadvantaged urban mothers in Canada: a mixed methods approach. Int J Behav Nutr Phys Act 2012;9:42.

40. Gyurcsik NC, Brawley LR, Spink KS, et al. Physical activity in women with arthritis: examining perceived barriers and self-regulatory efficacy to cope. Arthritis Rheum 2009;61(8):1087–94.

41. Farran CJ, Staffileno BA, Gilley DW, et al. A lifestyle physical activity intervention for caregivers of persons with Alzheimer's disease. Am J Alzheimers Dis Other Demen 2008;23(2):132–42.

42. Ene H, McRae C, Schenkman M. Attitudes toward exercise following participation in an exercise intervention study. J Neurol Phys Ther 2011;35(1):34–40.

43. Zalewski KR, Dvorak L. Barriers to physical activity between adults with stroke and their care partners. Top Stroke Rehabil 2011;18(Suppl 1):666–75.

44. Rimmer JH, Wang E, Smith D. Barriers associated with exercise and community access for individuals with stroke. J Rehabil Res Dev 2008;45(2):315–22.

45. Whitehead S, Lavelle K. Older breast cancer survivors' views and preferences for physical activity. Qual Health Res 2009;19(7):894–906.

46. Rogers LQ, Courneya KS, Robbins KT, et al. Physical activity correlates and barriers in head and neck cancer patients. Support Care Cancer 2008;16(1):19–27.

47. Rosqvist E, Heikkinen E, Lyyra TM, et al. Factors affecting the increased risk of physical inactivity among older people with depressive symptoms. Scand J Med Sci Sports 2009;19(3):398–405.

48. Stroud N, Minahan C, Sabapathy S. The perceived benefits and barriers to exercise participation in persons with multiple sclerosis. Disabil Rehabil 2009; 31(26):2216–22.

49. Rantakokko M, Iwarsson S, Kauppinen M, et al. Quality of life and barriers in the urban outdoor environment in old age. J Am Geriatr Soc 2010;58(11):2154–9.

50. Kirchhoff AC, Elliott L, Schlichting JA, et al. Strategies for physical activity maintenance in African American women. Am J Health Behav 2008;32(5):517–24.

51. Bjornsdottir G, Arnadottir SA, Halldorsdottir S. Facilitators of and barriers to physical activity in retirement communities: experiences of older women in urban areas. Phys Ther 2012;92(4):551–62.

52. Buttery AK, Martin FC. Knowledge, attitudes and intentions about participation in physical activity of older post-acute hospital inpatients. Physiotherapy 2009; 95(3):192–8.

53. Casey D, De Civita M, Dasgupta K. Understanding physical activity facilitators and barriers during and following a supervised exercise programme in Type 2 diabetes: a qualitative study. Diabet Med 2010;27(1):79–84.

54. Rogers C, Keller C, Larkey LK. Perceived benefits of meditative movement in older adults. Geriatr Nurs 2010;31(1):37–51.

55. Dlugonski D, Joyce RJ, Motl RW. Meanings, motivations, and strategies for engaging in physical activity among women with multiple sclerosis. Disabil Rehabil 2012;34(25):2148–57.

56. Resnick B, Vogel A, Luisi D. Motivating minority older adults to exercise. Cultur Divers Ethnic Minor Psychol 2006;12(1):17–29.

57. Bopp M, Lattimore D, Wilcox S, et al. Understanding physical activity participation in members of an African American church: a qualitative study. Health Educ Res 2007;22(6):815–26.

Maximizing ADL Performance to Facilitate Aging in Place for People with Dementia

Carrie A. Ciro, PhD, OTR/L, FAOTA

KEYWORDS

- Activities of daily living • Alzheimer disease • Dementia • Assistive technology
- Aging in place

KEY POINTS

- Disability in activities of daily living (ADL) is an inevitable outcome for people with all types of dementia.
- Undiagnosed and untreated ADL disability results in increased caregiver burden and increased risk of institutionalization for the person with dementia.
- Screening tools and performance-based evaluations are available to identify disability early and monitor the progression of ADL function over time.
- Evidence-based interventions are available to prevent, minimize, and delay ADL disability in people with dementia.

INTRODUCTION

More than 5 million Americans are diagnosed with Alzheimer disease (AD) and related dementias with each experiencing a unique constellation of cognitive, motor, and psychological manifestations of their particular dementia type.[1] Common to all will be inevitable disability in their ability to perform the activities of daily living (ADL) required for independent living.[1] Basic ADL (B-ADL) is commonly defined as those most basic life skills constituting the ability to care for one's self, which includes bathing, dressing, toileting, eating, and grooming.[2] Instrumental ADL (I-ADL) refers to more complex life skills for managing family and home environment, which includes cooking, cleaning, and financial management.[2] Retention of ADL performance is associated with personal, familial, and financial benefits, such as increased quality of life, decreased caregiver burden, and reduced care costs, as well as societal benefits such as a reduction

Disclosure Statement: The author has nothing to disclose.
Department of Rehabilitation Sciences, University of Oklahoma Health Sciences Center, 1200 North Stonewall Avenue, Oklahoma City, OK 73117, USA
E-mail address: carrie-ciro@ouhsc.edu

in institutional rates largely paid by national health programs.[1,3] Because of the negative impact of ADL disability on families and society, the importance of early detection and treatment of ADL disability, which when successful supports aging in place, deserves significant attention during the evaluation of older adults. Older adults with progressive neurologic processes such as dementia also require repeated monitoring and intervention as abilities change.[3,4]

To understand what types of ADL evaluation and intervention may be helpful, it must be understood how ADL is affected by the process of dementia. As dementia progresses, salient changes regarding ADL performance are observable and, in fact, are used to stage severity of dementia.[5–7] As an example, the progression of ADL disability as AD advances is illustrated in **Fig. 1**. The prodromal stage of AD, known as mild cognitive impairment, is diagnostically characterized as having only minor problems in I-ADL.[5,8] Specifically, changes in the quality of performance and timing of completion are noted with complex I-ADL, such as financial and medication management.[9] In mild cognitive impairment, no B-ADL changes are anticipated.[5,8] As the person moves into mild AD, disability in I-ADL is more obvious, as demonstrated by the need for support to complete complex tasks, such as cooking large meals or balancing the checkbook. Although B-ADL is largely intact, changes in the quality and frequency are reported.[1,3,10] For example, the person with mild AD may bathe less regularly and, when they do, they are likely less thorough than before the diagnosis. Moderate AD is demarcated by significant loss in both B-ADL and I-ADL.

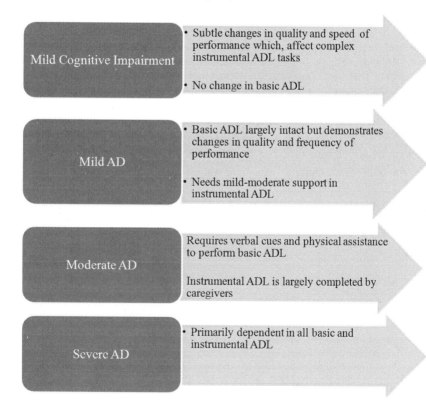

AD= Alzheimer's disease; ADL=activities of daily living

Fig. 1. Key indicators of ADL performance as Alzheimer disease progresses.

Progressive changes result in the need for verbal cues to initiate, sustain, and complete B-ADL, while the caregiver is primarily managing all I-IADL tasks. In severe AD, the person needs maximal to total assistance to complete all B-IADL and I-ADL.[1,3,10] Armed with understanding ADL changes in dementia, the clinician can begin to choose appropriate evaluations for each level of involvement.

EVALUATION OF ADL

Evaluation for the risk and presence of ADL disability is critical for supporting aging in place for people with dementia.[3,4,9] A variety of clinical tools are available to capture information about ADL performance, although one might argue that health professionals lack adeptness at discriminately using those tools, the consequence of which is inaccurate or biased results about ADL performance in people with dementia.[3] To improve accuracy and discrimination with ADL evaluation, the purpose of ADL screening versus ADL assessment is outlined in the context of facilitating aging in place, as well as methods used by each technique to capture information, pros and cons of each level of evaluation, and examples of clinical tools, which can be readily applied in most environments (**Table 1**).

ADL Screening

In the context of facilitating aging in place, the purpose of ADL screening is to determine risk or presence of ADL disability, as well as to monitor ADL function over time so that interventions can be initiated in a timely manner. Methods of ADL screening typically rely on questionnaires using self-informant or proxy-informants whereby the person is given simple response formats for the presence or absence of disability (eg, 1 = independence, 2 = some assistance needed, 3 = disability).[3,8] As an example, the Barthel Index of ADL is a 10-item scale that screens for disability in B-IADL and functional mobility (eg, transfers, mobility, and stairs).[11] Popular among clinicians, the Lawton IADL Scale is an 8-item scale that screens for performance in I-ADL and includes questions for phone use, shopping, food preparation,

Table 1
ADL evaluation in the context of facilitating aging in place: purpose, methods, and examples

Level of Evaluation	Purpose	Methods	Pros	Cons	Example of Clinical Tools
Screen	Is there a problem? Determine risk or presence of disability to ascertain service needs	Questionnaires Informant: • Self • Proxy	Quick and easy to administer Requires little training	Reliability decreases as informant self-awareness decreases or caregiver burden increases	Barthel Index of ADL Lawton-Brody IADL Scale
Assessment	What are the specifics of the problem? Determine specific plan of care for ADL	Performance-based observations of ADL performance	Reliable Garners specific information on impairments and function	Time-consuming Requires advanced training	Functional Independence Measure Performance Assessment of Self-Care Skills

housekeeping, laundry, medications, and finance management.[12] Both public domain tools can be administered to a patient or a proxy and are interpreted similarly whereby a lower total score indicates greater disability.[11,12] Neither tool indicates an absolute level of performance, which implies that someone could live alone safely, nor are they sensitive to the specific problems causing the dysfunction (eg, memory or motor function). Both the Barthel index and the Lawton scale are quick, easy to administer, require little training, and can be repeated at intervals to monitor gross function over time.

Despite the benefits of ease in using screening tools, biases inherent to self-report or informant-report scales affect the reliability of the screening scores for some patients. One bias lies in the lack of sensitivity of the scales. Most questionnaires, including the Barthel and Lawton tools, afford simple responses that do not include the best-matched level of performance for higher-functioning people.[8] For example, the person with mild cognitive impairment who has problems with quality or speed of performance will likely judge themselves as "independent" in a task instead of "needs assistance" or "dependent." An inaccuracy such as this creates a missed opportunity for intervention to facilitate aging in place for a person who is high functioning in early stages of dementia and presents with mild I-ADL disability.

A second common problem with screening tools is informant bias, which occurs because of error in reporting by either the person with dementia or their proxy. People with dementia have varying levels of self-awareness about their limitations, which typically results in *underreporting* problems with ADL and, if relied on, missed opportunities for interventions to facilitate aging in place.[5,8,13] Therefore, the accuracy of the person's estimation of their abilities must be measured before relying on self-report of functional ability.[14,15] Self-awareness can be measured in tools that examine the construct of self-awareness or by examining congruence with patient and caregiver scores on the same measure.[15] Depending on the setting, either method is useful and necessary to obtain an accurate screening. To add to the problem of self-informant bias, caregiver responses are influenced by the amount of burden they feel in relation to caring for the person with dementia.[13,16] Caregivers that report higher burden tend to exaggerate or *overreport* ADL disability by reporting higher assistance levels than are actually present. Overreporting ADL disability may result in the screener incorrectly advising the caregiver about potential for ADL recovery or recommendations for more supportive assistance than would be good for the person with dementia. For example, if a caregiver reports that their loved one needs total assistance for bathing and the person with dementia really needs minimal cues to initiate and complete bathing, a home health aide might be recommended for support instead of an occupational therapist for training to maximize bathing function.

ADL Assessment

The natural progression of ADL evaluation should be to first screen for disability and then perform an in-depth assessment of identified problem areas. As the next step to screening, performance-based assessments rely on observation to establish disability levels.[13,17] Through observation of the problem task, health professionals are able to identify specific problem areas that contribute to the disability and then determine a plan of care based on the results. For example, the Lawton IADL Scale would identify that a person has difficulty using a phone and a performance-based assessment would identify that disability in using the phone is caused by an inability to remember phone numbers and sequence the steps of making a phone call. Understanding factors that underlie the disability is necessary to create specific interventions that facilitate aging in place for people with dementia.[17,18]

As with screening tools, examples of ADL assessments are numerous. Commonly used tools in occupational therapy include the Functional Independence Measure (FIM) and the Performance Assessment of Self-Care Skills (PASS).[19,20] The FIM instrument is widely used in rehabilitation settings to determine the level of assistance needed to complete a variety of functional tasks, which include both B-ADL and I-ADL. Observation of performance is graded on a 7-point scale, where 1 = total assistance and 7 = independence. The evaluator is able to gauge the need for physical assistance, verbal assistance, or assistive technology alone. Observing performance at this level allows the examiner to see deficits in performance and provide tailored treatment plans for remediation or compensation.

Similarly, the PASS instrument allows the examiner to observe and rate B-ADL and I-ADL in the individual domains of independence, safety, and outcome (efficiency and accuracy) using a 3-point scale.[19,20] This distinction is very important, particularly for people with high-level cognitive deficits. For example, someone with mild cognitive impairment may be able to "independently" and "safely" cook a piece of chicken on the stove, but on cutting it at the table, may find that it is still raw, which is an "outcome" error. In pilot work, the author was able to discriminate between normal controls and people with mild cognitive impairment who presented with the type of subtle I-ADL disability described above using the PASS. In the context of aging in place, this is an important finding relevant for early identification of disability. Both tools are sensitive to changes due to intervention (eg, rehabilitation therapy or medications) and can be used to measure change over time.[20-22]

The benefit of performance-based testing includes greater reliability, sensitivity for identifying specific problem areas of ADL disability, and predictive abilities.[21,22] Problems with performance-based assessments include the need for advanced training and certification to administer most scales and the time-consuming nature of the assessment.[17] In summary, the ability to support aging in place for people with dementia is predicated on the ability to identify accurately risk and the presence of ADL disability so that appropriate services can be initiated to prevent, slow, or minimize loss of function. Judicious use and choice of ADL evaluation is recommended to discriminate the need for ADL intervention.

INTERVENTION

Once ADL disability is identified, evidence-based interventions for maximizing ADL performance should be initiated to facilitate aging in place. Although competing approaches can be found in literature, the intervention with the most promise for improving ADL performance in people with dementia is *task-oriented training*.[23,24] Task-oriented training uses real-life objects to train performance in contextually appropriate settings to regain lost skills. **Fig. 2** is an example of an interventionist working on improving cooking skills by practicing the specific skills needed to cook (preparing soup and muffins) according to the patient's diet and food preparation preferences. Practicing the ADL skills that are impaired draws on the strength of procedural long-term memory (unconscious memory for how tasks are done), which remains intact longer than declarative memory (conscious memory for names, facts) in people with dementia.[25,26]

Tasks chosen for training should be prioritized based on client and family goals. Facilitating individualized selection of goals allows the client and family to prioritize behavioral manifestations of dementia that cause the most distress given family resources.[18,27,28] It also allows the client to assert individual and family preferences (cultural values, gender preferences) within the context of social and environmental

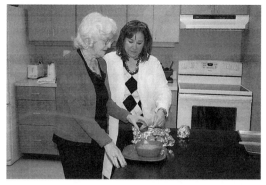

Fig. 2. Practicing cooking through task-specific training.

barriers and facilitators.[29] Client-chosen and family-chosen goals enhance motivation and the cooperative spirit between the interventionist and the family. An increasing number of studies are prioritizing personal goals to develop meaningful interventions in people with dementia.[18,27,30,31] Londos and colleagues[27] used the Canadian Occupation Performance Measure to illicit individual goals before teaching memory strategies to a sample with mild cognitive impairment. These goals were used to refine and individualize the memory strategies used in training. Statistically significant improvement in performance and satisfaction with performance after the intervention were maintained at the 6-month follow-up. Researchers using intervention strategies that focus on caregiver-identified goals have also shown decreases in negative client behaviors, improvements in functional performance, and decreased caregiver stress.[30–32]

In best practice, task-oriented training is planned using client-centered and family-centered goals with delivery of the intervention occurring through evidence-based training techniques of (1) development and maintenance of a therapeutic relationship; (2) repetitive, errorless learning (EL); (3) assistive technology; (4) cognitive strategies specific to ADL deficit; and (5) enhanced caregiver training with an emphasis on skill transfer (**Fig. 3**).

Therapeutic Relationship

Facilitating a therapeutic relationship with the person and their family is a central aspect of any therapeutic process and is considered as much an agent of change as the intervention itself.[33,34] It is not enough to simply include family goals in an intervention, the interventionist must enter the world of the participant, engage them socially and personally, earn their trust and respect, and work collaboratively with them to prioritize and work toward their goals.[34] Empathetic responses and actions demonstrate engagement and genuine belief in the person with whom you are establishing a relationship and signals that their participation is worth their effort during the intervention.[33,34] To facilitate aging in place for people with dementia, caregivers must be willing to understand the emotional, social, and financial issues that may work to displace them from their homes and maximize their trust to improve engagement in the process.

Repetitive, Errorless Training

EL is a training technique whereby the interventionist eliminates or reduces incorrect responses while teaching a new skill. Clare and Jones[35] suggest that EL can be achieved in a variety of ways to include (1) breaking tasks down into small, practicable

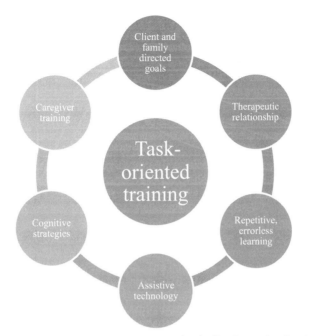

Fig. 3. Evidence-based intervention and structure for facilitating aging in place in people with dementia. Task-oriented training appears to be the most successful approach to improving ADL/IADL in people with dementia. The technique is enhanced by choosing goals for training that are based on client/family need, establishment of a therapeutic relationship with the client and family, delivering the intervention repetitively and free of error, using assistive technology and cognitive strategies, and using caregiver training techniques to enhance successful carry-over of therapeutic gains.

chunks and then repeating them in sequential order; (2) educating the person to avoid guessing; (3) preventing errors before occurring and correcting unintended errors immediately; and (4) modeling the task without errors before patient performance. Although simplistic in theory, EL is reinforced by neural processes that support new learning.[28,36] Current neuroscience suggests that neural connections are associated with specific experiences.[26] Dysfunctional practice may then lead to hardwiring the errors achieved in practice, particularly in a population that largely does not recognize their own errors for independent correction.[35,36] Although EL may feel intuitively correct, the existing evidence for EL supports use in practice. Although some studies have shown no advantage to using EL compared with errorful learning in people with early-stage dementia, a meta-analysis of EL intervention in patients with memory problems produced a large effect size of 0.87 when compared with patients that did not receive EL.[37]

Errorless learning appears useful for training daily life skills, particularly when paired with mass practice.[37] Mass practice schedules with high intensity, frequency, and duration of therapy appear to maximize rehabilitation potential in people with progressive and nonprogressive neurologic conditions.[38,39] In the author's work, she has examined dosage schedules equivalent to 3 h/d, 5 d/wk for 2 weeks in people with mild to moderate dementia, which has resulted in improved ADL performance and no increases in negative neuropsychological behaviors such as agitation or anxiety.[40] Offering opportunities for repetitive practice while minimizing errors during practice may be an important intervention strategy for maximizing ADL performance to support aging in place.

Cognitive Strategies

Cognitive strategies are methods of improving performance that either are directed by the individual (internal) or require external support (external). Internal strategies require that a person is aware of their limitation, is willing to use a strategy to overcome their limitation, and is able to remember the appropriate strategy at the appropriate time.[41] Therefore, internal strategies are used primarily with people with good self-awareness and high motivation to perform better. An example of an internal strategy is teaching a person with mild dementia with a visual processing problem to find the power button on a complex remote control by telling them to "feel for the top right button." External strategies are outside supports to function that may be initiated by the individual (eg, use of a day planner) or are preset by caregivers (eg, watch or medication alarms) and as a general rule include all forms of assistive technology discussed in the next section. External strategies can be successful in people with both mild and moderate dementia.[18,42–44] In the remote control example above, an external strategy for finding the power button might be changing the color or texture of the button so that it stands out among the rest. Examples of cognitive strategies useful for maximizing ADL are outlined in **Table 2**.[41,42,45,46] When delivered in the context of task-oriented training, the cognitive strategies chosen are specific to the task and the initiation of the strategy is blended in with the steps of the task so that task training seamlessly includes the chosen adaptations. Cognitive strategies play an important role in supporting ADL performance in older adults that are aging in place.

Assistive Technology

Because of the expansion and interest in new biomedical technologies, assistive devices to support older adult independence are growing in number, complexity, and usability. Devices can be used that not only monitor health status changes such as blood pressure, but data are now sent to physician offices for interpretation and early intervention.[47,48] Smart homes use voice recognition technology, which allows the user to turn on lights, adjust air temperature, or call emergency services from anywhere in the home.[47] Assistive technologies that support specific ADL tasks are widely available and are seen as mainstream advances versus assistance for people with disability.[47] For example, the use of medication organizers or medication alarms in watches can be used to remind people to take their medications, whereas electronic day planners within smart phones can be used to organize daily schedules. Popular, low-tech environmental modifications, such as grab bars and bath chairs, also support standing and transfer performance.[49]

Although research supports the use assistive technology for people with mild to moderate dementia, training or supports should vary by dementia stage.[42] For example, a person with mild dementia may be trained to incorporate and initiate a new strategy in a daily routine, such as using a day planner. However, a person with moderate dementia can be trained to only respond appropriately to an alarm that has been preset for their performance. To facilitate aging in place for people with dementia, a broad awareness of assistive technologies and the methods for incorporating them into ADL is useful.

Caregiver Training

Caregiver training is an important element for not only reducing caregiver burden but also improving patient performance outcomes. Caregiver training approaches that

Table 2
Common ADL errors, cognitive strategies, and technology to support intervention for aging in place

Common ADL Errors	Cognitive Strategies	Technology or Tools
Does not initiate ADL	Provide audio or visual external cues to initiate specific tasks identified as important.	Alarm, bell, timer, written list. Phone call from caregiver.
Decreased attention during ADL	Encourage eye contact on task.	Auditory alarm to cue back to task (bell).
	Search for information in a planned way (eg, left to right).	Bookmarker held in position on page to block extraneous information.
	Remove distractions or add music to keep focused.	Earplugs, MP3 music player.
	You have __ minutes to complete __.	Timer
Impaired visual processing for ADL	Encourage verbalizing what one is looking for before task (I am looking for the power button).	—
	Search for information in a planned way (eg, left to right).	Organize visual materials either independently or via caregiver.
	Highlight important items with color; make it bigger, or add more light.	Colored markers, Hi-Mark-TM tactile pen (Maxi-Aids, Farmingdale, NY, USA), task light, magnifying glass, or tools with built-in magnification (mirror). Large print. Increase space between lines.
Impaired memory for ADL	Use external strategies to prompt in weak areas.	Day planner, photo phone, medication alarm systems, and pill organizers.
Loses commonly used objects	Choose a location to store specific item.	Train to use "dumping stations" on entry to home, such as hanging key holders, or baskets.
	When possible have multiple sets of item (eg, keys, remote control).	
Problems sequencing ADL	Simplify the sequence by removing complex steps.	—
	Collect items needed for task before starting, which eliminates some steps.	—
	Check work against written list after each step; checking the step off the list reinforces the step was done.	Check-off list.
	Provide written, verbal, or tactile cues to move through steps.	Written list of steps. Audio play-by-play of steps using Step by Step Communicator (DynaVox Mayer-Johnson, Pittsburgh, PA, USA).
Difficulty organizing ADL	Preorganize before beginning (eg, get out items needed to make a sandwich).	Written list of steps.
	Simplify area; remove excess distractors.	Environmental modifications (eg, baskets, organizing trays for cabinets and drawers).

emphasize caregiver problem-solving and hands-on training reduce anxiety and feelings of burden in caregivers living with people with moderate to severe dementia.[30,31] Imperative to teaching new information to people with dementia is teaching the caregiver how to continue training when not in the presence of the interventionist. Training the caregiver to perform the intervention provides more repetition than can occur by the interventionist alone. Training also provides the caregiver with greater opportunity to explore the success of the intervention and empowers the caregiver to become part of the intervention team. Recent work on collaborative memory also suggests that training the caregiver and the client at the same time supports a spirit of working together to achieve a goal and a *collaborative memory*, which is recalled collectively when performing a task together, such as setting the table.[50] Clearly, caregiver training provides benefit for the client, caregiver, and the interventionist and provides additional value to interventions aimed at improving functional performance.

FUTURE DIRECTIONS

The most innovative changes in ADL evaluation and treatment will embrace technological advancements. Body sensors that can provide feedback about balance and strength during tasks, as well as the efficiency of performance (time to perform task, accuracy of task performance), are possible now and could be used to gauge ADL performance.[51–53] Home monitoring systems that video-record certain aspects of daily living available now could be used for monitoring and intervening to improve ADL performance for health teams in the future.[53] Exploring nonhuman assistance in the home is emerging in the literature in the form of robotic-assisted and animal-assisted models. Robots that can communicate socially have been tested in people with dementia and produce positive changes in sleep and cognition.[54,55] Animal-assisted models are emerging as a way to manage stress, behavioral outbursts, and functional performance issues.[56] Practitioners working with older adults should frequently update their knowledge of new technologies to provide cutting-edge treatments for adults with goals to age in their homes.

SUMMARY

Facilitating aging in place for people with dementia requires diligent monitoring of ADL function and early, as well as episodic, intervention for disability. Although disability may not be eliminated in people with dementia, minimizing the disruption of disability impacts caregiver burden and the potential to delay or prevent institutionalization. Interdisciplinary team management of ADL disability is arguably ideal for all settings that manage the care of older adults.

REFERENCES

1. Thies W, Bleiler L. 2011 Alzheimer's disease facts and figures. Alzheimers Dement 2011;7(2):208–44.
2. Moyers PA. The guide to occupational therapy practice. American Occupational Therapy Association. Am J Occup Ther 1999;53(3):247–322.
3. Desai AK, Grossberg GT, Sheth DN. Activities of daily living in patients with dementia: clinical relevance, methods of assessment and effects of treatment. CNS Drugs 2004;18(13):853–75.
4. Luck T, Luppa M, Wiese B, et al. Prediction of incident dementia: impact of impairment in instrumental activities of daily living and mild cognitive

impairment-results from the German study on ageing, cognition, and dementia in primary care patients. Am J Geriatr Psychiatry 2012;20(11):943–54.

5. Albert MS, DeKosky ST, Dickson D, et al. The diagnosis of mild cognitive impairment due to Alzheimer's disease: recommendations from the National Institute on Aging-Alzheimer's Association workgroups on diagnostic guidelines for Alzheimer's disease. Alzheimers Dement 2011;7(3):270–9.

6. McKhann GM, Knopman DS, Chertkow H, et al. The diagnosis of dementia due to Alzheimer's disease: recommendations from the National Institute on Aging-Alzheimer's Association workgroups on diagnostic guidelines for Alzheimer's disease. Alzheimers Dement 2011;7(3):263–9.

7. Burton CL, Strauss E, Bunce D, et al. Functional abilities in older adults with mild cognitive impairment. Gerontology 2009;55(5):570–81.

8. Winblad B, Palmer K, Kivipelto M, et al. Mild cognitive impairment—beyond controversies, towards a consensus: report of the International Working Group on Mild Cognitive Impairment. J Intern Med 2004;256(3):240–6.

9. Gold DA. An examination of instrumental activities of daily living assessment in older adults and mild cognitive impairment. J Clin Exp Neuropsychol 2012; 34(1):11–34.

10. Gillette-Guyonnet S, Andrieu S, Nourhashemi F, et al. Long-term progression of Alzheimer's disease in patients under antidementia drugs. Alzheimers Dement 2011;7(6):579–92.

11. Mahoney FI, Barthel DW. Functional evaluation: the Barthel index. Md State Med J 1965;14:61–5.

12. Lawton MP, Brody EM. Assessment of older people: self-maintaining and instrumental activities of daily living. Gerontologist 1969;9(3):179–86.

13. Schneider LS. Assessing outcomes in Alzheimer disease. Alzheimer Dis Assoc Disord 2001;15(Suppl 1):S8–18.

14. Banks S, Weintraub S. Self-awareness and self-monitoring of cognitive and behavioral deficits in behavioral variant frontotemporal dementia, primary progressive aphasia and probable Alzheimer's disease. Brain Cogn 2008;67(1): 58–68.

15. Snow AL, Norris MP, Doody R, et al. Dementia deficits scale. rating self-awareness of deficits. Alzheimer Dis Assoc Disord 2004;18(1):22–31.

16. Loewenstein DA, Argüelles S, Bravo M, et al. Caregivers' judgments of the functional abilities of the Alzheimer's disease patient. J Gerontol B Psychol Sci Soc Sci 2001;56(2):P78–84.

17. Goldberg TE, Koppel J, Keehlisen L, et al. Performance-based measures of everyday function in mild cognitive impairment. Am J Psychiatry 2010;167(7): 845–53.

18. Clare L, Linden DE, Woods RT, et al. Goal-oriented cognitive rehabilitation for people with early-stage Alzheimer disease: a single-blind randomized controlled trial of clinical efficacy. Am J Geriatr Psychiatry 2010;18(10):928–39.

19. Rogers JC, Holm MB, Beach S, et al. Task independence, safety, and adequacy among nondisabled and osteoarthritis-disabled older women. Arthritis Rheum 2001;45(5):410–8.

20. Rogers JC, Holm MB, Goldstein G, et al. Stability and change in functional assessment of patients with geropsychiatric disorders. Am J Occup Ther 1994;48(10):914–8.

21. Chumney D, Nollinger K, Shesko K, et al. Ability of functional independence measure to accurately predict functional outcome of stroke-specific population: systematic review. J Rehabil Res Dev 2010;47(1):17–29.

22. Peron EP, Gray SL, Hanlon JT. Medication use and functional status decline in older adults; a narrative review. Am J Geriatr Pharmacother 2011;9(6):378–91.

23. Arya KN, Pandian S, Verma R, et al. Movement therapy induced neural reorganization and motor recovery in stroke: a review. J Bodyw Mov Ther 2011;15(4): 528–37.

24. French B, Thomas LH, Leathley MJ, et al. Repetitive task training for improving functional ability after stroke. Cochrane Database Syst Rev 2007;(4):CD006073.

25. Li R, Liu KP. The use of errorless learning strategies for patients with Alzheimer's disease: a literature review. Int J Rehabil Res 2012;35(4):292–8.

26. Krakauer JW, Mazzoni P, Ghazizadeh A, et al. Generalization of motor learning depends on the history of prior action. PLoS Biol 2006;4(10):e316.

27. Londos E, Boschian K, Linden A, et al. Effects of a goal-oriented rehabilitation program in mild cognitive impairment: a pilot study. Am J Alzheimers Dis Other Demen 2008;23(2):177–83.

28. Jean L, Bergeron ME, Thivierge S, et al. Cognitive intervention programs for individuals with mild cognitive impairment: systematic review of the literature. Am J Geriatr Psychiatry 2010;18(4):281–96.

29. Sackett D, Straus S, Richardson W, et al. Evidence-based medicine: how to practice and teach EBM. 2nd edition. London: Churchill Livingston; 2000.

30. Gitlin LN, Corcoran M, Winter L, et al. A randomized, controlled trial of a home environmental intervention: effect on efficacy and upset in caregivers and on daily function of persons with dementia. Gerontologist 2001;41(1):4–14.

31. Gitlin LN, Winter L, Vause Earland T, et al. The Tailored Activity Program to reduce behavioral symptoms in individuals with dementia: feasibility, acceptability, and replication potential. Gerontologist 2009;49(3):428–39.

32. Chee YK, Gitlin LN, Dennis MP, et al. Predictors of adherence to a skill-building intervention in dementia caregivers. J Gerontol A Biol Sci Med Sci 2007;6(6): 673–8.

33. Norcross JC, Wampold BE. Evidence-based therapy relationships: research conclusions and clinical practices. Psychotherapy 2011;48(1):98–102.

34. Peloquin SM. The patient-therapist relationship in occupational therapy: understanding visions and images. Am J Occup Ther 1990;44(1):13–21.

35. Clare L, Jones R. Errorless learning in the rehabilitation of memory impairment: a critical review. Neuropsychol Rev 2008;18(1):1–23.

36. Jean L, Simard M, van Reekum R, et al. Towards a cognitive stimulation program using an errorless learning paradigm in amnestic mild cognitive impairment. Neuropsychiatr Dis Treat 2007;3(6):975–85.

37. Kessels RP, de Haan EH. Implicit learning in memory rehabilitation: a meta-analysis on errorless learning and vanishing cues methods. J Clin Exp Neuropsychol 2003;25(6):805–14.

38. McIntyre A, Viana R, Janzen S, et al. Systematic review and meta-analysis of constraint-induced movement therapy in the hemiparetic upper extremity more than six months post stroke. Top Stroke Rehabil 2012;19(6):499–513.

39. Peurala SH, Kantanen MP, Sjogren T, et al. Effectiveness of constraint-induced movement therapy on activity and participation after stroke: a systematic review and meta-analysis of randomized controlled trials. Clin Rehabil 2012;26(3): 209–23.

40. Ciro C, Hershey L, Garrison D. Enhanced task-oriented training in a person with dementia with Lewy-bodies. Am J Occup Ther 2013;67:556–63.

41. Toglia J, Goverover Y, Johnston MV, et al. Application of the multicontextual approach in promoting learning and transfer of strategy use in an individual

with TBI and executive dysfunction. OTJR (Thorofare N J) 2011;31(Suppl 1): S53–60.

42. Bourgeois MS, Camp C, Rose M, et al. A comparison of training strategies to enhance use of external aids by persons with dementia. J Commun Disord 2003;36(5):361–78.
43. Bourgeois MS, Dijkstra K, Burgio L, et al. Memory aids as an augmentative and alternative communication strategy for nursing home residents with dementia. Augment Altern Commun 2001;17(3):196–210.
44. Clare L, van Paasschen J, Evans SJ, et al. Goal-oriented cognitive rehabilitation for an individual with Mild Cognitive Impairment: behavioural and neuroimaging outcomes. Neurocase 2009;15(4):318–31.
45. Padilla R. Effectiveness of environment-based interventions for people with Alzheimer's disease and related dementias. Am J Occup Ther 2011;65(5):514–22.
46. Letts L, Edwards M, Berenyi J, et al. Using occupations to improve quality of life, health and wellness, and client and caregiver satisfaction for people with Alzheimer's disease and related dementias. Am J Occup Ther 2011;65(5):497–504.
47. Brandt A, Samuelsson K, Toytari O, et al. Activity and participation, quality of life and user satisfaction outcomes of environmental control systems and smart home technology: a systematic review. Disabil Rehabil Assist Technol 2011; 6(3):189–206.
48. Dewsbury G, Linskell J. Smart home technology for safety and functional independence: the UK experience. NeuroRehabilitation 2011;28(3):249–60.
49. Korp KE, Taylor JM, Nelson DL. Bathing area safety and lower extremity functions in community-dwelling older adults. OTJR (Thorofare N J) 2012;32(2):22–9.
50. Neely AS, Vikström S, Josephsson S. Collaborative memory intervention in dementia: caregiver participation matters. Neuropsychol Rehabil 2009;19(5): 696–715.
51. Bankole A, Anderson M, Smith-Jackson T, et al. Validation of noninvasive body sensor network technology in the detection of agitation in dementia. Am J Alzheimers Dis Other Demen 2012;27(5):346–54.
52. Bergmann JH, Smith IC, Mayagoitia RE. Using a body sensor network to measure the effect of fatigue on stair climbing performance. Physiol Meas 2012; 33(2):287–96.
53. Darwish A, Hassanien AE. Wearable and implantable wireless sensor network solutions for healthcare monitoring. Sensors (Basel) 2011;11(6):5561–95.
54. Moyle W, Cooke M, Beattie E, et al. Exploring the effect of companion robots on emotional expression in older adults with dementia: a pilot randomized controlled trial. J Gerontol Nurs 2013;39(5):46–53.
55. Tanaka M, Ishii A, Yamano E, et al. Effect of a human-type communication robot on cognitive function in elderly women living alone. Med Sci Monit 2012;18(9): CR550–7.
56. Filan SL, Llewellyn-Jones RH. Animal-assisted therapy for dementia: a review of the literature. Int Psychogeriatr 2006;18(4):597–611.

The Older Adult with Diabetes
Peripheral Neuropathy and Walking for Health

Elena Cuaderes, PhD, RN[a],*, W. Lyndon Lamb, DPM[b],
Anne Alger, BSN, RN[c]

KEYWORDS

- Aging • Walking • Diabetes mellitus • Risk for foot ulcers • Risk for falling
- Prevention

KEY POINTS

- Diabetic peripheral neuropathy can lead to infected ulcers and necessitate nontraumatic amputation of lower limbs. It can also increase the risk for falling.
- Walking is the preferred method of exercise for most older people and helps individuals with diabetes mellitus (DM) to achieve and maintain euglycemia.
- If preventive measures and behaviors are not practiced as recommended, walking can lead to foot trauma and injurious falls.
- With the client as the center of the team, services from a variety of health care specialist are required to prevent foot ulcers and injurious falls in the aging adult with DM.

INTRODUCTION

A nurse is working in the primary care clinic when Ms Johnson, an older person with long-duration type 2 diabetes, comes in for her quarterly visit. Even though the patient insists that there is no pain or discomfort, you have observed a stage 3 ulcer on the first metatarsal head of her right foot. The patient's history reveals diabetic retinopathy and sensorimotor peripheral neuropathy. Ms Johnson notes that she has a new walking partner and feels compelled to go along with the plan that this person has suggested. Her walking partner insists that their daily morning walks be longer and further than what the patient is used to. The patient also speaks of an injurious fall that she

Disclosure: The authors have nothing to disclose.
[a] Academic Programs, College of Nursing, University of Oklahoma Health Sciences Center, 1100 North Stonewall Avenue, Oklahoma City, OK 73117, USA; [b] Podiatry, Choctaw Nation Health Care Center, One Choctaw Way, Talihina, OK 74571, USA; [c] Cardiac Care, OU Medical Center, 700 Northeast 13th Street, Oklahoma City, OK 73104, USA
* Corresponding author.
E-mail address: elena-cuaderes@ouhsc.edu

experienced a few weeks ago while walking in a crowded shopping mall. This incident required a visit to the emergency department.

The scenario presented here is a common one in clinics where persons with diabetes are treated. The rate at which diabetes mellitus (DM) is being diagnosed in adults aged 65 to 79 years continues to increase. According to the Centers for Disease Control and Prevention (CDC), this incidence rate per 1000 people increased from 10.3 in 1997 to 12.5 in 2010.[1] The American Diabetes Association (ADA) claims that there are now 10.9 million people more than 65 years of age with this potentially serious disease.[2] These facts increase concern about the ability of older, active individuals with DM to remain healthy and to successfully age in place. One way to remain healthy and prevent the complications of diabetes is to regularly exercise,[3] and according to Belza[4] walking seems to be the method preferred by most older individuals, regardless of ethnicity. However, walking under pathologic conditions arising from peripheral neuropathy (PN) is known to contribute to foot trauma that leads to ulcers and ultimately infection and amputation. PN can also lead to balance problems, placing the individual at risk for fall injuries.[5]

Ulcer prevention in people with DM and PN focuses on early detection of trauma to the lower extremities. The incidence of foot ulcers in those with DM is estimated to be up to 25%,[6] and they are costly.[7] It has been noted that 1 in 3 adults, 65 years of age or older, have had falls yearly and 20% to 30% of these cases result in moderate to severe injuries.[5] Both situations tend to rob a person of independent living and progress the client toward a path to early death.

HOW DOES PN DEVELOP?

The most common complication of both type 1 and type 2 DM is PN, which is known to occur primarily as a result of long duration and persistent hyperglycemia.[8] Recent studies have shown that, although effective glycemic control seems to be the primary factor in preventing PN in those with type 1 DM, this may not be the case in people with type 2 DM.[9] Obesity, hypertension, dyslipidemia, inflammation, and insulin resistance may contribute as much as hyperglycemia to the development of PN.

The prevailing hypothesis, although not entirely understood, speculates that multiple abnormal metabolic processes, as a result of hyperglycemia and impaired insulin receptor signaling, lead to an oxidative stress that exceeds the antioxidant capacity of the body.[10] Excess reactive oxygen species (metabolic byproducts), mediated by a reduction in nitric oxide, damage the endothelium of blood vessels that supply the nerves. With an ensuing nerve hypoxia, cells that are responsible for the health of the myelin and axons are injured and demyelination and axon damage result. It is the axon injury that is responsible for the loss of protective sensation (LOPS), loss of tendon reflexes, and muscle wasting of the lower limb. In addition, the nonenzymatic glycation (the covalent bonding of glucose to proteins or lipids without the action of an enzyme) of soft tissue and bone protein is thought to lead to collagen abnormalities that leave the foot and ankle with cheiroarthropathy (limited joint mobility) because of thickening of the skin, tendons, ligaments, and joint capsules.[11] Despite higher bone mass densities from nonenzymatic glycation, individuals with type 2 DM tend to have higher rates of hip and wrist fractures.[12]

HOW DOES NEUROPATHY LEAD TO DIABETIC FOOT ULCERS?

The tendency for foot and ankle abnormalities from PN is primarily based on an interrelationship of changes to the sensory, motor, and autonomic nerve systems. Neuropathy typically starts with an abnormality of the sensory system and evolves in a bilateral, symmetric, and stockinglike pattern of distribution, meaning that symptoms such as tingling and numbness start at the toes and progress proximally toward the feet and legs.[8] Because sensory nerves allow the detection of pain, light touch, vibration, and temperature discrimination, LOPS of the foot increases the risk for undetected injury. Those affected characteristically report stepping on a sharp object with the bare foot or sustaining a friction wound from ill-fitting shoes, both of which can lead to ulcers and infection. Some degree of sensation loss is present in 30% of those with DM who are more than 40 years old.[13] Furthermore, substances from the unmyelinated C-fibers that modulate inflammation are rendered dysfunctional by sensory neuropathy, resulting in impaired inflammatory responses.[14] These reduced responses increase the risk of persons not recognizing the warning signs of pain or redness caused by trauma or infection. It is possible for this dysfunction to cause people to have the inability to detect inflammation of the feet, even after repetitive walking, thus increasing the risk for ulcer formation. Charcot joint (**Fig. 1**), described by the American Orthopaedic Foot and Ankle Society,[15] is a condition that mostly affects adults with DM, aged 40 years and older, and can result from the stress of repetitive walking on a severely insensate limb. It is usually characterized by noninfectious, single or multiple joint dislocations or fractures, and destruction of the foot architecture. Unless properly treated, it too can lead to ulceration and amputation.

Motor axons tend to be more resistant to the effects of DM than sensory axons, and the signs and symptoms of their injury usually appear later in the disease process. However, when it occurs, patients present with impaired mobility because of lower limb muscle wasting, weakness, and disfigurement. Often called the intrinsic minus foot, this condition refers to the lumbricals of the foot, which are the first muscles of the lower limb to be affected by damage to the motor nerves.[16] Weakness of these muscles leads to toe and foot deformities.

Autonomic neuropathy (AN), when severe, usually results in a global anhidrosis (diminished or absent sweating) and this initial loss of normal thermoregulatory sweating proceeds in a stocking pattern in the lower limbs.[17] As a result, patients experience dryness of the feet that contributes to the formation of cracks and fissures.

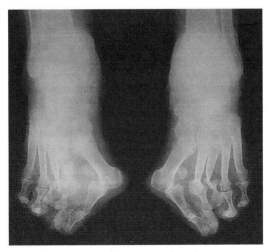

Fig. 1. Charcot joint. (Biophoto Assoc./Photo Researchers.)

These skin breaks expose the bare foot to microorganisms that can later be hard to eradicate within the diabetic vascular environment. With ischemia from vascular damage, bacterial invasion, and an existing reduction in immune defenses, a nonhealing wound and amputation may soon follow. Along with diabetes-related sensorimotor neuropathy, anhidrosis, extrinsic factors such as ill-fitting shoes, and foot and ankle deformities, add to the physical stresses of walking and can result in callus formation of the plantar foot.[18,19] Calluses, which have been shown to increase foot-floor contact (plantar pressures), have consistently been associated with ulcer formation and tend to occur mostly at the first, second, and third metatarsal heads (**Fig. 2**) and hallux (great toe).[20] According to experts,[11,21] diabetic foot wounds are primarily a product of 3 situational events, related to walking, that can result in foot wounds.

Peripheral arterial disease (PAD), although not a key factor in the development of diabetic foot lesions, is a major feature in the nonhealing ulcer and it accounts for at least 60% of all foot wounds.[22] Because of the distinctive structure of the cutaneous microcirculation of the feet, a pattern emerges that describes capillary basement membrane thickening, a loss of vasoconstrictor tone, arteriovenous shunting, and increases in tissue pressures. In addition, occlusive narrowing from macrovascular atherosclerosis develops. Therefore, less oxygen and nutrients are available to the lower limb and, as a result, ischemia develops (**Fig. 3**).[14,21,22] Furthermore, neuropathy tends to blunt the pain of claudication.[23] With this situation, patients tend to present to their health care providers later and with more severe cases of this condition. Analyzed data from male veterans who were diabetic and aged 30 to 85 years showed that, of the 8 most frequent pathways that accounted for 73% of all diabetic amputations, 4 of these pathways indicated that foot trauma led to ulceration, faulty healing, infection,

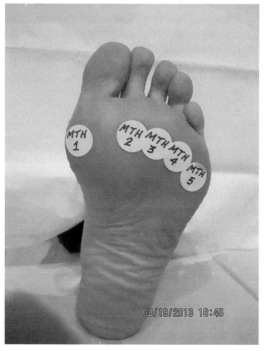

Fig. 2. Location of metatarsal heads (MTH) 1 to 5 on the plantar foot.

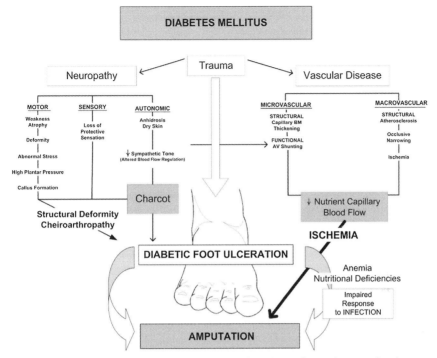

Fig. 3. The major factors in the development of diabetic foot ulcers and subsequent amputation. (*Reprinted from* Frykberg RG, Zgonis T, Armstrong DG, et al. Diabetic foot disorders. A clinical practice guideline (2006 revision). J Foot Ankle Surg 2006;45(Suppl 5): S-6; with permission from Elsevier.)

and ultimately gangrene.[24] Preceding all 4 of these pathways was a report of lower limb ischemia and sensory neuropathy.

HOW DOES NEUROPATHY LEAD TO A RISK FOR FALLS?

Maintaining balance requires a complex system of sensory inputs and motor outputs.[25] It has been reported that fall risk, either with standing or walking, is substantially increased when individuals with DM have diminished sensation of the feet and weak dorsiflexor muscle strength, which reduces the ability to rapidly develop torque about the ankle.[26] Therefore, individuals tend to compensate for deficits by walking slower, taking shorter strides, and spending more time in the double support phase of the gait cycle. In addition, if a person has not adapted to a surface that is irregular and not smooth, fall risk may be greater. Adding to these limitations is recent evidence that shows that the odds of having vestibular dysfunction are increased in individuals with PN[27] and, according to an expert panel,[28] retinopathy is strongly associated with it as well. Given these shortcomings, fall risk is increased because balance primarily is achieved through input to the brain from the eyes and the vestibular system, and a sense of position is achieved with intact sensory nerves as well as output from the brain to the muscles that control lower limb movement.[25] With differences in balance ability, walking speed, and endurance, people with PAD and DM show significantly lower extremity function than people with PAD and no DM.[29]

WHAT DO I NEED TO KNOW ABOUT EXAMINING THE FOOT AND ASSESSING THE RISK FOR FALLS?

A thorough foot examination cannot be performed unless Ms Johnson's shoes and socks have been removed and the lighting in the examination room is adequate. The most basic assessment maneuver for patients at risk is one that tests for LOPS. Evidence shows that the 10 g Semmes-Weinstein monofilament is one of the most effective screening tools to use in the clinical setting.[30] A recent systematic review revealed that at least 3 sites should be tested to detect PN as early as possible and the most commonly recommended sites are the plantar aspect of the hallux, and the first, third, and fifth metatarsal heads.[31] This method is quick, painless, and inexpensive and should be used each time the foot is examined by the clinician. Although there remains controversy about the use of the monofilament as the sole instrument to test for LOPS, the ADA recommends the use of additional tests such as vibration sense and temperature perception in order to increase the sensitivity for detecting PN.[32] Ask Ms Johnson whether she has been experiencing pain, burning, tingling, and numbness of the feet. These symptoms are typically the first to be experienced and they indicate small fiber neuropathy.[33] The gold standard of testing modalities, a nerve conduction study, is usually negative in early PN because this test serves to measure abnormalities of the large fibers.

Motor neuropathy is associated with the loss of ankle reflexes with cheiroarthropathy of the foot and ankle and is especially seen in individuals with a history of ulcers. A goniometer is the standard tool for measuring the degree of dorsiflexion at Ms Johnson's ankle and an absent reflex is determined by placing it in a neutral position before striking the stretched Achilles tendon with the percussion hammer.[32] On observation and palpation of her foot, an intrinsic minus foot is identified by such things as hammer toes, distal migration of the metatarsal fat pads resulting in prominent metatarsal heads, weak extension of the hallux, and a high arch from the tightening of the plantar fascia.[16] All of these features can result in wounds of the foot through ill-fitting footwear and repetitive stress from walking.

Charcot joint typically affects the midfoot and, on examination, is unilateral, erythematous, warm, and swollen.[15,34] This condition should immediately be referred to a podiatrist or other specialist for care. In addition, if Ms Johnson shows some degree of PAD, along with PN, she is especially prone to toenail onychomycosis (fungal infection). This condition occurs because of her immune, vascular, and neurologic status and possible faulty walking biomechanics.[35] Not only can this condition cause embarrassment for her but she may have difficulties in walking and problems with proper shoe fit as well. At present, and depending on the extent of the problem, topical and systemic medications are available for treatment.[36] The most common form of onychomycosis is characterized by nail thickening, yellow discoloration, and sometimes detachment of the nail plate from the nail bed.[35] Measuring temperature differences at a site on one foot and comparing it with the same site of the other foot with an infrared dermal thermometer may be useful in helping individuals modify their walking activity. It has been suggested that temperature differences of greater than 2.2°C are an indication that individuals with DM, an ulcer history, and some degree of PAD should lessen their weight-bearing activity and should not resume their normal pattern of walking until these differences are less than this point.[37]

A foot affected by AN presents with sudomotor (sweat gland nerve fibers) dysfunction. Check Ms Johnson for anhidrosis of the feet. It usually is most prominently seen at the heels and, if there is also callus formation at these sites, both combine to increase the risk of deep fissure formation.[19] A plantar foot callus in a person without neuropathy is painful and off-loading typically facilitates healing of the lesion. However, in a person with neuropathy and no perceived pain from the callus while walking, repetitive pressure continues and injury occurs.[18] Therefore, it is vital that the feet are examined for calluses and fissures. AN can be a problem for the ambulating individual if signs and symptoms of unstable cardiovascular and respiratory systems are present. Exercise intolerance can manifest as decreased heart rate variability, exercise orthostasis and hypotension, and impaired ventilator reflexes.[38] It is recommended that exercise testing be undertaken for individuals who have suspected or known cardiac AN and who wish to start a program of walking.[3,39]

A primary assessment maneuver for vascular sufficiency in Ms Johnson is the determination of a pulse at the posterior tibial and dorsalis pedis sites.[32] If there is no pulse, an ankle-brachial index (ABI) pressure should be obtained. The ABI is measured by dividing the ankle systolic pressure by the brachial systolic pressure; any value that is 0.8 or less indicates insufficiency. The ABI can be falsely increased in DM because of medial calcinosis (calcium deposits).[32] It has recently been discovered that the toe-brachial index may be a better indicator of the extent of PAD in the distal extremities because arteries of the digits are less affected by calcinosis.[40] If Ms Johnson has a history of smoking, previous ulcers, amputation, Charcot joint, claudication, angioplasty, vascular surgery, diabetic retinopathy, and nephropathy, then she is at very high risk for developing ulcers of the foot.[32]

Simple, inexpensive, and quick patient-initiated maneuvers and tools are available to assess Ms Johnson's balance and risk for falling. The timed-up-and-go test, the standing unassisted test, and the Tinetti Mobility Scale were found to be adequate screening measures among older individuals.[41] Fall risk from neuropathy can also be determined by establishing the degree of lower extremity weakness and loss of sensation, presence of comorbidities such as arthritis, and the use of certain medications.[41,42] Also, knowing whether there is a past-year history of falls, with or without injury, is vital.

WHAT SHOULD I TELL THE CLIENT ABOUT PREVENTION OF FOOT ULCERS AND FALLING?

A cornerstone of preventing ulcers is foot care.[43] Ms Johnson needs to know that daily visualization for lesions on the top and bottom of each foot, careful washing, and drying and moisturizing the feet are necessary. Also, she needs to be informed about preventing exposure of her feet to heat and cold, and about trimming toenails. If physical limitations prevent her from adequately observing and reaching the foot, a mirror or family assistance may be necessary. The foot specialist may recommend that toenail cutting be performed by a professional only. It has been shown that 23% to 63% of people with DM rarely or never check their feet.[44] Education may not be sufficient to induce behavior changes and it seems that it only produces short-term results.[45] Nonetheless, it is important that patients understand the information, are motivated to perform the tasks, and possess the ability to perform these skills. Investigators found that a longer duration of the patient-provider relationship increased adherence to daily foot checks.[46] Another group discovered that, if information was easily remembered by the client, there was a greater likelihood of daily foot care behavior.[47]

It is recommended that, in order to prevent ulcers, Ms Johnson should at least have semiannual foot examinations if she has LOPS.[21] She should also consider appropriate footwear according to the characteristics of the foot.[6] Calluses should be debrided by a specialist.[21] Although well-fitting walking or athletic shoes are appropriate for those with only neuropathy and increased plantar pressures, custom-molded shoes are necessary for people with bony deformities such as Charcot foot. The ADA recently changed its stance on weight-bearing exercise (ie, walking) and PN and now recommends that moderate-intensity walking is appropriate.[3]

After a formal gait assessment by a specialist, Ms Johnson may need to be encouraged to use an assistive device with advice from an occupational therapist, or she may need to undergo a program of strength and balance training.[42] Walking is a good way to help achieve and maintain glycemic control and it is advised, if the person is able, to perform a minimum of 150 minutes per week of moderate-intensity exercise.[3] Because a foot lesion has been detected on Ms Johnson's foot, it should be offloaded and non–weight-bearing exercise performed.

SUMMARY

Complications from diabetic PN can prevent Ms Johnson from healthy aging in place, and health maintenance for people like her requires extensive management from the individual and the health care team. Identifying those at increased risk for debilitating foot ulcers and falls generally are referred to the primary care clinician.[6] However, a care team comprising of case managers, dieticians, advanced nurse practitioners, nurse educators, physical therapists, and physicians should ideally be in place to provide holistic care. Patients with negative attitudes and poor resources should be referred to the appropriate professionals for ongoing support and reinforcement of interventions.

Foot ulcers, amputations, and a risk for falls are the result of many factors that can be categorized as molecular, anatomic, and environmental influences. For instance, hyperglycemia leads to the production of reactive oxygen species, which results in an anatomic change to the nerve blood vessels, leaving the person with LOPS. LOPS poses a risk if the environment is one that the person cannot tolerate. Changes of the motor nerves from hypoxic damage lead to lower limb insensation, muscle atrophy, and weakness. With impaired sensory input and motor output, the person is prone to injurious falls, especially if environmental influences, such as a throw rug on the floor, contribute. Despite improvements in glycemic control in persons with diabetes in recent years,[48] scientists continue to test novel therapies that act to prevent neuropathies of diabetes. Such agents include alpha lipoic acid to scavenge reactive oxygen species,[49] aminoguanidine to prevent nonenzymatic glycation,[50] and neuritin to regenerate axons.[51]

REFERENCES

1. CDC. Diabetes data and trends [website]. 2011. Available at: http://www.cdc. gov/diabetes/statistics/incidence/fig5.htm. Accessed July 29, 2013.
2. ADA. Diabetes basics. 2013. Available at: http://www.diabetes.org/diabetes-basics/diabetes-statistics/. Accessed July 29, 2013.
3. American Diabetes Association. Standards of medical care in diabetes–2013. Diabetes Care 2013;36(Suppl 1):S11–66.
4. Belza B, Walwick J, Shiu-Thornton S, et al. Older adult perspectives on physical activity and exercise: voices from multiple cultures. Prev Chronic Dis 2004;1(4): A09.
5. CDC. Costs of falls among older adults. Injury and violence prevention and control: home and recreational safety [Web page]. 2010. Available at: http://www. cdc.gov/HomeandRecreationalSafety/Falls/fallcost.html. Accessed June 9, 2011.

6. Singh N, Armstrong DG, Lipsky BA. Preventing foot ulcers in patients with diabetes. JAMA 2005;293(2):217–28.
7. Kitsnet RS. The standard of care for evaluation and treatment of diabetic foot ulcers. 2010. Available at: https://www.barry.edu/includes/docs/continuing-medical-education/diabetic.pdf. Accessed March 6, 2014.
8. Tesfaye S, Selvarajah D. Advances in the epidemiology, pathogenesis and management of diabetic peripheral neuropathy. Diabetes Metab Res Rev 2012; 28(Suppl 1):8–14.
9. Callaghan BC, Hur J, Feldman EL. Diabetic neuropathy: one disease or two? Curr Opin Neurol 2012;25(5):536–41.
10. Dobretsov M, Romanovsky D, Stimers JR. Early diabetic neuropathy: triggers and mechanisms. World J Gastroenterol 2007;13(2):175–91.
11. van Schie C, Slim FJ. Biomechanics of the diabetic foot: the road to foot ulceration. In: Veves A, Giurini JM, LoGerfo FW, editors. The diabetic foot. New York: Humana Press; 2012. p. 203–16.
12. Hofbauer LC, Brueck CC, Singh SK, et al. Osteoporosis in patients with diabetes mellitus. J Bone Miner Res 2007;22(9):1317–28.
13. CDC. 2011 National diabetes fact sheet. 2011. Available at: http://www.cdc.gov/diabetes/pubs/factsheet11.htm. Accessed July 29, 2013.
14. Richard JL, Lavigne JP, Sotto A. Diabetes and foot infection: more than double trouble. Diabetes Metab Res Rev 2012;28(Suppl 1):46–53.
15. AOFAS. Charcot joints or neuropathic arthropathy. 2013. Available at: http://www.aofas.org/footcaremd/conditions/diabetic-foot/Pages/Charcot-Joints-or-Neuropathic-Arthropathy.aspx. Accessed July 29, 2013.
16. Bernstein RK. Physical signs of the intrinsic minus foot. Diabetes Care 2003; 26(6):1945–6.
17. Freeman R. Autonomic peripheral neuropathy. Neurol Clin 2007;25(1):277–301.
18. Mueller MJ, Maluf KS. Tissue adaptation to physical stress: a proposed "Physical Stress Theory" to guide physical therapist practice, education, and research. Phys Ther 2002;82(4):383–403.
19. Pavicic T, Korting HC. Xerosis and callus formation as a key to the diabetic foot syndrome: dermatologic view of the problem and its management. J Dtsch Dermatol Ges 2006;4(11):935–41.
20. Bus SA, Maas M, de Lange A, et al. Elevated plantar pressures in neuropathic diabetic patients with claw/hammer toe deformity. J Biomech 2005;38(9): 1918–25.
21. Frykberg RG, Zgonis T, Armstrong DG, et al. Diabetic foot disorders. A clinical practice guideline (2006 revision). J Foot Ankle Surg 2006;45(Suppl 5):S1–66 [Update of J Foot Ankle Surg 2000;39(Suppl 5):S1–60; PMID: 11280471].
22. Gibbons GW, Shaw PM. Diabetic vascular disease: characteristics of vascular disease unique to the diabetic patient. Semin Vasc Surg 2012;25(2): 89–92.
23. American Diabetes Association. Peripheral arterial disease in people with diabetes. Diabetes Care 2003;26(12):3333–41.
24. Pecoraro RE, Reiber GE, Burgess EM. Pathways to diabetic limb amputation. Basis for prevention. Diabetes Care 1990;13(5):513–21.
25. VDA. The human balance system: good balance is often taken for granted. 2013. Available at: http://vestibular.org/understanding-vestibular-disorder/human-balance-system. Accessed March 6, 2014.
26. Macgilchrist C, Paul L, Ellis BM, et al. Lower-limb risk factors for falls in people with diabetes mellitus. Diabet Med 2010;27(2):162–8.

27. Agrawal Y, Carey JP, Della Santina CC, et al. Diabetes, vestibular dysfunction, and falls: analyses from the National Health and Nutrition Examination Survey. Otol Neurotol 2010;31(9):1445–50.

28. Tesfaye S, Boulton AJ, Dyck PJ, et al. Diabetic neuropathies: update on definitions, diagnostic criteria, estimation of severity, and treatments. Diabetes Care 2010;33(10):2285–93.

29. Dolan NC, Liu K, Criqui MH, et al. Peripheral artery disease, diabetes, and reduced lower extremity functioning. Diabetes Care 2002;25(1):113–20.

30. Feng Y, Schlosser FJ, Sumpio BE. The Semmes Weinstein monofilament examination as a screening tool for diabetic peripheral neuropathy. J Vasc Surg 2009; 50(3):675–82, 682.e1.

31. Dros J, Wewerinke A, Bindels PJ, et al. Accuracy of monofilament testing to diagnose peripheral neuropathy: a systematic review. Ann Fam Med 2009;7(6): 555–8.

32. Boulton AJ, Armstrong DG, Albert SF, et al. Comprehensive foot examination and risk assessment: a report of the task force of the Foot Care Interest Group of the American Diabetes Association, with endorsement by the American Association of Clinical Endocrinologists. Diabetes Care 2008;31(8):1679–85 [Reprints in J Am Podiatr Med Assoc 2009;99(1):74–80; PMID: 19216129; and Phys Ther 2008;88(11):1436–43; PMID: 19137633].

33. Tavee J, Zhou L. Small fiber neuropathy: a burning problem. Cleve Clin J Med 2009;76(5):297–305.

34. Rogers LC, Frykberg RG, Armstrong DG, et al. The Charcot foot in diabetes. Diabetes Care 2011;34(9):2123–9.

35. Thomas J, Jacobson GA, Narkowicz CK, et al. Toenail onychomycosis: an important global disease burden. J Clin Pharm Ther 2010;35(5):497–519.

36. Tosti A, Sche RK, Vinson RP, et al. Onychomycosis treatment & management. Medscape: drugs, diseases and procedures. 2013. Available at: http://emedicine. medscape.com/article/1105828-treatment. Accessed August 5, 2013.

37. Lavery LA, Higgins KR, Lanctot DR, et al. Preventing diabetic foot ulcer recurrence in high-risk patients: use of temperature monitoring as a self-assessment tool. Diabetes Care 2007;30(1):14–20.

38. Albright A. Exercise precautions and recommendations for patients with autonomic neuropathy. Diabetes Spectrum 1998;11(4):231–7.

39. Pop-Busui R. Cardiac autonomic neuropathy in diabetes: a clinical perspective. Diabetes Care 2010;33(2):434–41.

40. Bonham PA. Get the LEAD out: noninvasive assessment for lower extremity arterial disease using ankle brachial index and toe brachial index measurements. J Wound Ostomy Continence Nurs 2006;33(1):30–41.

41. Thurman DJ, Stevens JA, Rao JK. Practice parameter: assessing patients in a neurology practice for risk of falls (an evidence-based review): report of the Quality Standards Subcommittee of the American Academy of Neurology. Neurology 2008;70(6):473–9.

42. Rubenstein LZ. Falls in older people: epidemiology, risk factors and strategies for prevention. Age Ageing 2006;35(Suppl 2):ii37–41.

43. ADA. Living with diabetes: foot care. 2013. Available at: http://www.diabetes.org/ living-with-diabetes/complications/foot-complications/foot-care.html. Accessed July 30, 2013.

44. McInnes A, Jeffcoate W, Vileikyte L, et al. Foot care education in patients with diabetes at low risk of complications: a consensus statement. Diabet Med 2011;28(2):162–7.

45. Dorresteijn JA, Kriegsman DM, Assendelft WJ, et al. Patient education for preventing diabetic foot ulceration. Cochrane Database Syst Rev 2012;(10):CD001488.
46. Piette JD, Schillinger D, Potter MB, et al. Dimensions of patient-provider communication and diabetes self-care in an ethnically diverse population. J Gen Intern Med 2003;18(8):624–33.
47. Bundesmann R, Kaplowitz SA. Provider communication and patient participation in diabetes self-care. Patient Educ Couns 2011;85(2):143–7.
48. Hoerger TJ, Segel JE, Gregg EW, et al. Is glycemic control improving in U.S. adults? Diabetes Care 2008;31(1):81–6.
49. Shay KP, Moreau RF, Smith EJ, et al. Alpha-lipoic acid as a dietary supplement: molecular mechanisms and therapeutic potential. Biochim Biophys Acta 2009; 1790(10):1149–60.
50. Thornalley PJ. Use of aminoguanidine (Pimagedine) to prevent the formation of advanced glycation endproducts. Arch Biochem Biophys 2003;419(1):31–40.
51. Karamoysoyli E, Burnand RC, Tomlinson DR, et al. Neuritin mediates nerve growth factor–induced axonal regeneration and is deficient in experimental diabetic neuropathy. Diabetes 2008;57(1):181–9.

Medication Adherence in Older Adults

The Pillbox Half Full

Kathy Henley Haugh, PhD, RN, CNE

KEYWORDS

- Medication adherence • Older adults • Aged • Medication interventions
- Reminder systems

KEY POINTS

- Medication nonadherence is a common concern for nurses and family members who care for older adults.
- Understanding the reason for nonadherence is essential in achieving the desired clinical and behavioral outcomes.
- Traditional interventions, such as educational and behavioral interventions, must often be combined to be successful.
- New technologies offer nurses opportunities to explore interventions for the baby boomers, who are now tapping into Medicare.

Drugs don't work in patients who don't take them.[1(p487)]
—*C. Everett Koop, MD, former Surgeon General.*

Nurses and family members are often perplexed at finding a patient or loved one's pillbox still half-full at the end of the week. What are the reasons for medication nonadherence? What strategies can support adherence to taking medications, especially in older adults? Nurses need to appreciate and address adherence concerns for the present population of older adults, and nurses need to be proactive in researching ways to help baby boomers to adhere to medication regimens. Baby boomers officially became Medicare beneficiaries in 2011. The purpose of this article is to explore the reasons for medication nonadherence, research the literature for interventions that have demonstrated effectiveness in improving adherence, provide a framework for organizing and applying this knowledge, review research for new directions, and conclude with implications for nursing practice and research.

The author has nothing to disclose.
Acute and Specialty Care, University of Virginia School of Nursing, 225 Jeanette Lancaster Way, PO Box 800826, Charlottesville, VA 22908-0826, USA
E-mail address: khh@virginia.edu

NONADHERENCE AS A PREVALENT AND COSTLY PROBLEM

The 2008 national population projections estimated that there were 40.2 million Americans aged 65 and older in 2010; this number is projected to rise to 88.5 million older adults in 2050.[2] Between 2000 and 2002, a typical patient receiving Medicare saw a median of 7 physicians per year, 2 for primary care and an additional 5 specialists.[3] This creates the potential for older adults to have numerous prescriptions, with the potential for duplications and unintended interactions. In a survey of medication use in 3500 community-residing older adults (age 57–87 years), researchers found that 81% of respondents reported having 1 medication prescription, with 29% reporting a total of 5 or more prescriptions.[4]

Data suggest that 50% of patients with chronic illnesses do not take medications as prescribed, with 20% to 30% of prescriptions never even filled.[5–7] In older adults, systematic reviews cite nonadherence as between 40% and 75%, cautiously noting that this large range reflects the variety of methods used to measure adherence as well as the effects of different illnesses, medications, and settings.[8,9] The financial costs of nonadherence is staggering, estimated from $289 billion[1,7] to $310 billion annually.[7] The Centers for Disease Control and Prevention reports the human toll of nonadherence to cause between 30% and 50% of treatment failures and 125,000 deaths annually.[5,10]

DEFINITIONS

The World Health Organization (WHO) defines adherence as "the extent to which a person's behavior—taking medication, following a diet, and/or executing lifestyle changes, corresponds with agreed recommendations from a health care provider."[11(p3)] The Agency for Healthcare Research and Quality (AHRQ) defined medication adherence as "the extent to which patients take medication as prescribed by their health care providers."[7(p1)] The AHRQ and an International Society for Pharmacoeconomics and Outcomes Research Medication Compliance and Persistence working group distinguish between medication adherence and medication persistence. *Medication adherence* relates to the timing, dosage, and frequency in the day-to-day routine; *medication persistence* relates to the consistency in taking a prescribed medication for a prescribed length of time.[7]

INTENTIONAL VERSUS UNINTENTIONAL NONADHERENCE

One consideration when discussing adherence is differentiating between intentional and unintentional nonadherence.[12] *Intentional nonadherence* is an individual's premeditated decision to not take a medication. A patient may even choose not to fill a prescription, as discussed previously; this is termed *primary nonadherence*. Intentional nonadherence may occur because of an individual's belief system, such as a belief that medications are overprescribed. Intentional nonadherence may also occur based on an individual's analysis of the risk-versus-benefit profile, such as side effects outweighing perceived benefit from the medicine. In either case, the individual is specifically choosing to not take the medication. *Unintentional nonadherence* arises when an individual fully intends to take a medication but fails to do so for a variety of reasons, including most often forgetfulness. Other barriers include expense, transportation concerns, and even physical constraints, such as vision and dexterity.

Some health care providers might label intentional nonadherence a compliance issue, which tends to assign blame to patients. Osterberg and Blaschke[1] first used the AHRQ definition of medication adherence interchangeably for both medication adherence and compliance, lamenting the imperfections that exist using either term. In a majority of recent literature, medication adherence is the term most consistently used to infer the collaborative versus passive role of consumers/patients. Nurses and health care professionals need to understand the reason for nonadherence to tailor interventions that are effective to the cause. For a more detailed discussion of intentional and unintentional medication nonadherence, readers are referred to Lehane and McCarthy.[13]

WHAT INTERVENTIONS HAVE PROVED EFFECTIVE?

In 2008 and 2009, several quality reviews were published specific to medication adherence. An updated Cochrane review[6] analyzed 79 short-term and long-term randomized controlled trials (RCTs). Short-term treatments were included if they successfully followed participants in 80% of cases and long-term treatments had to have at least 6 months of follow-up. Five of the 10 short-term studies showed a positive effect on adherence, with 4 of the studies also showing improvement in at least one clinical outcome, such as blood pressure. Interventions that helped short-term adherence included counseling, providing written information, and making personal phones calls. Of the 81 interventions evaluated in the long-term studies, 25 led to an improvement in a clinical outcome and 36 produced an improvement in adherence. Interventions included instructions to the patient (verbally, in writing, or visually), disease/therapy counseling, promoting empowerment, working with family members and other social support systems, peer mentoring, making therapy more convenient, automated or manual phone calls, computer-assisted monitoring, simplifying doses, providing reminders through daily habits, special packages for medications, dose-dispensing units/charts, direct observation of treatment, augmenting pharmacy services, and involving patients in some aspect of care (eg, blood pressure). Unfortunately, only studies that used a combination of interventions to promote long-term adherence showed a significant result. Only 2 of the studies in this particular Cochrane review addressed the complex regimens in the older adult population[14,15]; neither of these studies found an intervention of significance.

WHAT ABOUT OLDER ADULTS SPECIFICALLY?

A literature review[16] focused on older adults analyzed 63 studies published between 1977 and 2005. A criterion for inclusion in this review was a mean age of greater than 60 years. Interventions fell into 3 overall categories: patient-focused, medication or prescription focused, and interventions specific to actually taking the medication. Patient-focused interventions included patient education, written information, disease education, and interventions to train individuals on self-administration, motivational counseling, social support, and symptom self-monitoring. Interventions that focused on the medications or prescriptions included dose modification, packaging, and medication review. Interventions that focused on administering or taking the medications included reminders, such as calendars, charts, phone calls, postcards, and monitoring or tracking behavior. Only 3 of the 63 studies included family or caregivers in the study intervention. The investigators noted the prevalence of educational interventions within these 63 studies, suggesting the need to study more behavioral interventions (especially those related to forgetfulness), the role of significant others, and the role of the health care system itself (eg, access and costs).

That review of literature[16] presents an overview of the many interventions studied up until 2005. These same investigators and others followed their review of literature with a meta-analysis.[17] A meta-analysis applies statistical models to rigorously selected studies so that conclusions can be drawn from participants across a variety of studies. Using these advanced statistical concepts, an analysis of 11,827 older adult participants occurred across 33 studies conducted between 1970 and 2007. Interventions found the most effective included special medication packaging, dose modification, participant monitoring of side effects and medication effects (such as blood pressure), succinct written instructions, and standardized, versus tailored, approaches. These findings substantiate that a variety of educational and behavioral interventions can effectively increase medication adherence in older adults.

ARE THESE STUDIES MEANINGFUL?

Limitations to the literature to date include the following: inconsistent measures of adherence across studies, lack of clinical endpoints, complex/labor intensive interventions,[6] lack of generalizability,[6,16] and insufficient sample size.[6,17] Limitations also are acknowledged in the criteria for systematic review studies, for example, including only English language studies or RCT designs.[6,16,17]

In addition, there is a need to strengthen studies on adherence and be more holistic in addressing medication adherence by incorporating a theoretical foundation into future studies.[17,18] A discussion of such theories is beyond the scope of this article. Russell and colleagues,[19] however, provide a brief overview of 3 such theories that have relevance to medication adherence: Bandura's social cognitive theory,[20] Ajzen's and Fishbein's theory of planned behavior,[21] and Leventhal and colleagues' self-regulation model.[22] These investigators concluded that there is a need for a paradigm shift to a personal systems approach that focuses more on the individual in the environment. Building on the work of Alemi and colleagues[23] regarding continuous self-improvement and systems thinking, the investigators define personal systems change as "a process of systematically improving individual systems through collaboratively shaping routines, involving supportive others in routines, and using medication self-monitoring to change and maintain behavior."[19(p274)] Theories can help practitioners be holistic in researching the etiology of nonadherence and to know how to intervene more effectively.

HOW TO MEASURE ADHERENCE

The inconsistency in measuring adherence has been a concern in nonadherence research. The WHO[11] suggests that the state-of-the-art measurement for adherence should include both a subjective self-report measure and an objective measure of adherence. As such, nurses need to look for both subjective and objective measures in determining the quality of a research study, and nurses who design their own research studies need to include both measures of adherence.

Subjective measures most often include Morisky's 4-item self-report scale (**Box 1**)[24]; this scale and a longer 8-item Morisky scale have both reported validity in the literature.[24,25] In a study of 299 community-dwelling adults over 60 years of age, the following findings using Morisky's 4-item scale are revealing: 33% reported that they forget to take their medications; 10% reported being careless in taking their medicine; 7% said they had stopped taking their medicine when they felt better; and 11% stopped taking their medicine when they felt worse.[26] Researchers caution against interpreting all cases of forgetfulness and carelessness as unintentional; behaviors may actually be more intentional, related to unresolved concerns or beliefs about their medications.[27]

Objective measures often include biochemical measures (cholesterol levels and blood pressure) or electronic or computerized medication monitoring systems.[11,28]

Box 1
Morisky's 4-item self-report scale

1. Do you ever forget to take your medicine?

2. Are you careless at times about taking your medicine?

3. When you feel better, do you sometimes stop taking your medicine?

4. Sometimes if you feel worse when you take the medicine, do you stop taking it?

From Morisky DE, Green LW, Levine DM. Concurrent and predictive validity of a self-reported measure of medication adherence and long-term predictive validity of blood pressure control. Medical Care 1986; Morisky DE, Malotte CK, Choi P, et al. A patient education program to improve rate with antituberculosis drug regimens. Health Education Quarterly 1990;17:253–68; and Morisky DE, DiMatteo MR. Improving the measurement of self-reported medication nonadherence: Final response. J Clin Epidemio 2011;64:258–63. Use of the ©MMAS is protected by US copyright laws. Permission for use is required. A License agreement is available from: Donald E. Morisky, ScD, ScM, MSPH, Professor, Department of Community Health Sciences, UCLA School of Public Health, 650 Charles E. Young Drive South, Los Angeles, CA 90095-1772.

The Medication Event Monitoring System (MEMS)[29] has been widely used across studies. This device uses microelectronic circuits in the cap of the device to record the date and time that the medication container is opened and closed.

SEEING THE BIG PICTURE—THE WORLD HEALTH ORGANIZATION FRAMEWORK

A second major limitation of research studies has been the lack of a framework to organize or conceptualize the holistic nature of adherence.[17–19] With more than 200 variables cited as contributing to nonadherence, it is important that a health care team choose interventions that are appropriate to the cause of the nonadherence. One framework that acknowledges the breadth and depth of adherence is the WHO 5 dimensions model (**Fig. 1**).[11] This model cites the interrelationship of the following 5 dimensions to nonadherence: health system/health care team factors, social/economic factors, therapy-related factors, condition-related factors, and patient-related factors.

Health system/Health Care Team (HCT) factors include the knowledge and training of health care providers to educate patients, time for consultation, and the infrastructure—the red tape of health care. Social and economic factors may include having to make choices between medications and putting food on the table, illiteracy, transportation concerns, or the lack of a social support network. Condition-related factors include the symptoms and disability that threaten a patient's ability to be adherent. Therapy-related factors include the consequences of following a recommended therapy: the side effects, the scheduling, and the do's and don'ts associated with each medicine (with meals, on an empty stomach, and so forth). Patient-related factors range from forgetfulness, anxiety, poor eyesight, confidence, and motivation to beliefs about the inherent risk-benefit relationship of the therapy to deeper beliefs about health and illness in general. All of these dimensions are interrelated; all of these dimensions are patient centered.[11]

The WHO 5 dimensions model[11] provides a useful framework for reflecting on the big picture, thereby facilitating an assessment that is more holistic, uncovering all potential areas of concern where interventions might be helpful. Nurses can also use this model to categorize interventions for nonadherence (**Box 2**). Such organization can facilitate the tailoring of intervention(s) to the cause(s) for nonadherence. The interventions found in **Box 2** align with the 5 dimensions presented by the WHO and include

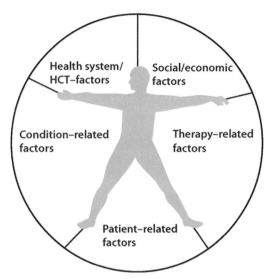

Fig. 1. The 5 dimensions of adherence. HCT, Health Care Team. (*From* Sabate E. Adherence to long-term therapies. Evidence for action. Geneva (Switzerland): World Health Organization; 2003. Available at: http://www.who.int/chp/knowledge/publications/adherence_report/en/index.html.)

interventions found in the literature reviews discussed previously. Perusing these 5 dimensions, nurses can identify areas for innovation as well as gaps in efforts to be holistic in intervening in medication nonadherence.

NEW DIRECTIONS: INNOVATIONS IN TECHNOLOGY

Electronic monitoring systems are often used in research to collect data as a measure of adherence. These devices, intended to facilitate data collection, were also observed to increase adherence. One analysis of 48 studies[30] found that coupling electronic medication-event monitoring methods with feedback to patients improved adherence by 19.8% compared with 10.3% in studies that did not use this type of feedback. The MEMS[29] unit was the pioneer objective measure of medication adherence. Since these early studies, electronic reminder systems have expanded in design and scope. Several products are now available to consumers. These devices are numerous and range in price from $9.95 to $844.95 depending on the features.[31] Products can be as simple as once-a-day pillboxes with alarms to tamper-proof automatic medication dispensers. Designs include watch alarms, pendants, electronic pillboxes, and electronic blister packs.

One promising area for nursing research and even product design incorporates computer technology to prescribe medication safely and to promote medication adherence among health care providers. Increasingly, health care providers use computerized decision-making support systems that provide significant prompts and reminders to effectively and safely prescribe medication and monitor for concerns. These systems have reported to be modestly effective in improving safety in prescription behaviors of health care providers.[9] Such technology is increasingly targeted to the consumers to promote adherence through devices, such as smartphones and personal computers. These interventions have been the focus of the more recent research.

These technologies are increasingly explored even with older adults. The use of mobile phone devices with older adults has been explored across clinical areas (eg, diabetes and palliative care), with aims ranging from exploring device feasibility and acceptability to the impact on patient care, such as memory enhancement, wandering safety in Alzheimer disease, fall detection, symptom reporting/monitoring in chronic illness, exercise logs/programs, and standardized provider responses to data entry by patients.[32] The importance of mobile phone design and education is emphasized as a major consideration when using this technology with older adults, given age-related changes in dexterity, vision, hearing, and even preference for familiar features, such as hardware buttons instead of touch screens. Further suggestions include research to address the frequency, method, and type of message alerts that are provided to patients, such as standardized alerts or alerts that require a patient to respond. In addition, the burden on providers with monitoring patient data entry is cited as a potential area of concern. Despite the relative newness of such research, some investigators are optimistic about the role of this technology in combating nonadherence: "[I]f system designers were to select a technology platform that would reach the majority of older adults, mobile phones would be ideal due to their high penetrance rate."[32(p947)]

One analysis of 11 studies included a variety of electronic reminders: pagers, interactive voice response systems, video-telephone calls, and programmed electronic audiovisual reminder devices in addition to mobile phone device reminders.[33] Overall the participants who received a reminder intervention using any of these devices demonstrated a significant increase in dose adherence (65.94% reminder groups and 54.71% control groups). Suggested limitations to these devices focused on practical considerations, such as projected cost-effectiveness of implementation (no data actually stated) and long-term feasibility. Other investigators agree with these limitations, noting that although evidence exists for these technological interventions in the short term (less than 6 months), the long-term effects are still unknown.[34] It is postulated that adults taking medication for chronic illnesses, such as glaucoma, HIV, asthma, and hypertension, might become immune to daily reminders; a weekly reminder may be just as effective. Such limitations reiterate the need to continue to use practical reminder-based interventions, such as blister packages and calendars; advantages may arise with newer technology with these more practical time-tested interventions.[33]

WILL OLDER ADULTS USE THE NEWER TECHNOLOGY?

Two of the 3 reviews discussed previously did not limit their analysis to older adults.[33,34] Therefore, the question remains, do (or will) older adults even use these devices? Perhaps, the more realistic question is, will the newly inducted generation of older adults, the baby boomers, use these devices? According to the Pew Research Center,[35] 56% of American adults now own a smartphone of some kind. Manufacturers are now making simplified smartphones with features that are specifically designed for older adults.[36] The implications for marketing are only increasing. Smartphone devices are already programmed to run health care–related applications (apps). In a recent review,[37] 160 smartphone apps were found that were designed specifically for medication adherence. Pharmacists ranked these apps, rating MyMedSchedule, MyMeds, and RxmindMe as the 3 top apps based on reminder features and the potential functions that they offer. Features included reminders not requiring Internet connections and the ability to track doses (electronically and in print). Approximately half of the apps are free, with the price of other apps averaging $2.83. One app

---

Box 2
Interventions for improving patient adherence using the WHO 5 dimensions

Social and economic factors

- Work with an interdisciplinary team (social worker, case manager, and so forth) to address the following issues: uninsured, underinsured, Medicare concerns, unemployed, copayments, homeless, lack of family/social support, transportation/driving safety, and scheduling.
- Learn about the costs of medications and suggest alternative less-expensive medications when alternatives do not affect clinical outcome.
- Provide educational materials based on health literacy level and patient's preferred language.
- Offer community peers as resources or advocates for patients when beliefs, cultures, or language concerns are present.
- Learn about age-specific resources and communicate these to patients (eg, MTM plans with Medicare).
- Learn about national and state policies that could increase patient adherence to medications. Advocate for policies that are consistent with your values. Be open to policies that conflict with your values.

Health system/health care team factors

- Advocate for continuity of care.
- Advocate for care coordinators to oversee recommendations from multiple providers/ specialists.
- Maintain a friendly, professional environment to decrease stress of patient visits. Consider the physical environment as well—walkers, wheelchairs, parking, lighting.
- Communicate! Use open-communication techniques that encourage questions, work for solutions, and do not place blame.
- Actively address institutional issues that affect patient adherence, such as time waiting for prescriptions. Call prescriptions into pharmacies to decrease wait times and to communicate special patient needs (see "Patient-related factors").
- Stay informed of interventional research on medication adherence.

Therapy-related factors

- Work with the interdisciplinary team to minimize complexity of regimen—once-a-day dosing, times consistent with patient routines, combination pills where possible, and simplicity/appropriateness of route of administration.
- For every new medication prescribed—use teach back to assure understanding and to identify barriers to implementation. Include purpose and rationale for medication, method of administration, administration guidelines (empty stomach), side effects, and duration of therapy. Determine work-around for barriers OR change medication if possible.
- Review medications with each visit to determine continued need.
- Work with the interdisciplinary team to minimize frequent/multiple changes in therapy.

Condition-related factors

- Work with interdisciplinary team to address comorbidities that affect adherence (stress reduction, alcohol, substance abuse, and depression).
- Again, work with the interdisciplinary team to minimize frequent/multiple changes in therapy and to coordinate services among primary care providers and specialists.

Patient-related factors

- Develop an individualized approach to adherence based on assessment of patient's unique barriers and resources. Include both educational and behavioral interventions.

- Work with the interdisciplinary team to address individual social and economic concerns, as noted previously (finances, cultural beliefs, health care beliefs, social stigma, and literacy)

- Work with the health care team and educational experts to design effective educational tools (written, auditory, and visual) appropriate to literacy level and cultural preference. Assure materials are easy to use, time effective, and appropriate to the unique needs of an older adult population, such as sensory impairments (vision and hearing).

- Provide additional resources based on assessment (eg, suggestions on appropriate Internet resources to explore).

- Notify pharmacists of visual impairments for labeling containers.

- Notify pharmacists of manual dexterity impairments for container options.

- Provide suggestions for patients that may address memory, forgetfulness, and need for routine:
  - Automated refill reminders
  - Pillboxes
  - Blister packages
  - Calendars
  - Homemade resources (modification of egg cartons or toolbox organizers)
  - Electronic medication monitoring systems
  - Automated dispensing systems
  - Daily routines (brushing teeth, meals, bedtime, and leaving for work)
  - Automated reminder messages (texting, phone calls, and beepers)
  - Personal reminder messages (significant others and daily visits)
  - Smartphone medication reminder applications
  - Community resources

- When providing suggestions to patients, determine feasibility and unintended consequences of presumably helpful suggestions (privacy, access to medications by others, and unintentional double dosing).

- Proactively work with patients who are concerned with potential side effects to learn how to recognize them, how to minimize them, and when to seek additional care.

- Proactively work with patients to incorporate medications into daily life to preserve quality of life (eg, diuretics).

- Where appropriate, have patient/support system monitor and record clinical outcomes for feedback (eg, blood pressure and blood glucose).

- Suggest community resources to build skills and confidence (community colleges, librarians, faith-based nurses, peer volunteers, and local agencies for seniors).

Adapted from Sabate E. Adherence to long-term therapies: evidence for action. Geneva (Switzerland): World Health Organization; 2003; and Centers for Disease Control and Prevention. Medication Adherence, CDC's Noon Conference. March 17, 2013. Available at: http://www.cdc.gov/primarycare/materials/medication/docs/medical-adherance-transcript.pdf.

(MyMeds) offers a companion Web site with an annual subscription fee of $5.99. The underlying expense can be a limiting factor. All smartphone devices with app potential require a phone purchase and monthly data plans.

One nursing study of 35 participants with chronic illness used simple handheld devices to deliver audible electronic beeps at the time medications were due.[38] Participants who completed the study achieved an 89.64% adherence rate, which was commendable. Of particular interest were the anecdotal data gathered on the 8 participants who did not complete the 12-week study (23% attrition rate). Reasons for not completing the study included the following: too much work, got in the way of life, left at home, remembering to use device was a hardship, not fun, and did not like it. Such reasons may translate to the use of mobile cellular devices and other technology being evaluated today.

The commercial world is increasingly responding to the market to be senior friendly. GreatCall[39] markets a Jitterbug cellular phone, advertised as more senior friendly with simpler interfaces, longer battery life, and features that are mindful of sensory impairment. The phone also features a 24-hours a day urgent response system and a medication app called MedCoach, for reminders and pharmacy interfaces. GreatCall service plans range from $15 to $80 per month with the purchase of the phone unit at $99 to $119.00. Other manufacturers are also creating simpler interfaces, for example, the Easy Mode option on the Samsung[40] Galaxy S 4 mobile phone.

Tablets are the more recent technological advance on the health care scene. According to a Pew Report, 18% of those 65 and older own a tablet.[41] A majority of tablet users, however, are ages 35 to 44 (49%), not the younger generations. Companies are already marketing computer tablets designed specifically for older adults. One such tablet is the Claris Companion.[42] These tablets can be programmed remotely from a caregiver's computer to include only those features needed by the older adult, simplifying its use. Features include large texts and buttons, amplified speakers, a large screen, and one-touch buttons to check in, send emails, or even view an exercise video (**Fig. 2**). Medication and event reminders are programmable as reminder alerts and can be monitored by a caregiver. Owning such a device costs

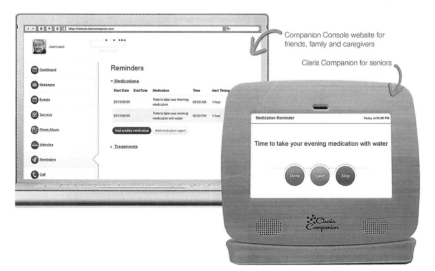

Fig. 2. Tablet technology for older adultd: the Claris Companion. (*Courtesy of* Claris Healthcare, Ferndale, WA; with permission.)

approximately $649 with monthly rates of $49 per month. The device is marketed as a simpler alternative to computers and laptops for older adults.

Systems that are more elaborate have also evolved. In the United Kingdom, an experiment known as Enhanced Complete Ambient Assistive Living Experiment uses smartphone technology to monitor patients in the home environment.[43] A smartphone app receives input from a "smart" garment with wireless health sensors that the older adult wears. A Global Positioning System sensor in the smartphone communicates with a remote server that is accessed by health care professionals. In 2011, researchers began exploring similar technology where the ingestion of pills can be remotely monitored by electrical impulses that are created from natural substances released when the pill is swallowed.[44]

Technology provides many new approaches to address nonadherence, and technology is attempting to be senior friendly. Within this growing maze of smart garments, smartphones, tablets, and texting technology, however, are embedded Health Insurance Portability and Accountability Act confidentiality issues as well as privacy issues and potential exploitation of patients.[37,43] Health care providers, researchers, and family members must remain vigilant as to what is in the best interest of patients or loved ones.

NEW DIRECTIONS: POLICY

Most recent literature remains focused on interventions aimed at patients, such as reminder systems and education. One systematic review purposefully sought to explore provider, systems, and policy interventions that were aimed to improve medication adherence.[7] Overall results were consistent with previous studies: a combination of education and behavioral interventions offers the most evidence of improvement. This review of 62 studies, however, also reported on positive results from case management for adults with diabetes, hypertension, heart failure, and depression. In addition, 9 studies were included that addressed policy interventions, all measuring adherence by the number of insurance claims for processing prescriptions. The interventions for each of these 9 studies decreased out-of-pocket expenses through reducing copayments or improving prescription drug coverage. Although results were inconsistent across studies, there was robust evidence to support that reduced out-of-pocket expenses improves medication adherence. The investigators further contend that such policy measures can benefit more individuals because these approaches are less complex, are less labor-intensive than many other interventions, and they can reach more patients geographically. The mean age of the participants in these studies was not provided; however, the focus of the studies was chronic illness. According to the American Hospital Association,[45] 60% of older adults will manage more than 1 chronic condition by 2030.

Since 2006, Medicare Part D providers have been required to offer a medication therapy management (MTM) plan for eligible beneficiaries.[46] Although implementation varies, the Centers for Medicare & Medicaid Services (CMS) provide guidelines for these plans.[46] Since 2013, everyone who is eligible must be offered a plan. To be eligible, an older adult should have between 2 and 3 chronic diseases, take 2 to 8 medications covered by Medicare Part D, and have estimated annual out-of-pocket expenses of $3144. The CMS requires programs to annually review all medications, prescription and otherwise, and prepare a written summary of that review within 2 weeks for patients, encouraging patients to share the review with their provider. Targeted quarterly reviews are then required. A study of Medicare beneficiaries in 2010 compared those with and without MTM plans.[47] Patients who were studied had either heart failure or chronic obstructive pulmonary disease. Results demonstrated that benefits of the plan often included an increased use of medications. The patients who also received comprehensive medication reviews had greater benefits. Limitations to analysis in this study included inconsistency in design, with extra services included by some organizations. Given the increased use of medications observed by those with MTM plans, however, nurses need to know to counsel patients as to the services offered from these plans; eligible gerontological nurse specialists may oversee these plans and bill Medicare accordingly.

As more nurses expand their roles into health policy, nurses need to advocate for policy measures to decrease out-of-pocket expenses for older adults. The Affordable Care Act[48] is currently in a state of flux as to the details of implementation; it cannot be known what the Affordable Care Act will mean for patients with chronic illness, especially the older adult population. Therefore, nurses must remain politically savvy and policy focused to influence these decisions.

NEW DIRECTIONS: CREATIVE SOLUTIONS, UNIQUE POPULATIONS

The need for research continues. In June of 2013, the Food and Drug Administration (FDA) announced the availability of funds to promote medication adherence in Americans: "[The] FDA is committed to addressing this issue, which has enormous implications for public health and the U.S. economy…"[49(p34109)]

New models of care should be explored as to their impact on medication adherence, for example, medical (health) homes. The URAC (an independent nonprofit accreditation organization) defines a patient-centered health care home as a "quality-driven, interdisciplinary, clinician-led team approach to delivering and coordinating care that puts patients, family members, and personal caregivers at the center of all decisions concerning the patient's health and wellness."[50(pp15–16)] Nurses can research the effect of medical health homes on medication adherence in older adults.

Older adults with special needs must be considered when considering best practice specific to medication adherence. Older adults with memory impairments present special challenges for nurses. In a clinical trial of 27 participants with memory impairment, interventions that included automated reminding and tailored information had higher levels of medication adherence than a control group.[51] In addition, the presence of a caregiver produced substantially higher levels of adherence. This is consistent with other studies that demonstrated frequent human communication along with reminder systems might be more appropriate for older adults with cognitive changes.[52]

Unique barriers in this population with memory impairments include understanding new directions, living alone, and establishing a routine. Routine can be a powerful intervention for older adults. In a study of 84 older adults,[53] mealtime, wake-up, and sleep routines were integrally involved in medication behaviors for 94% of the sample. Prompts included where the medication was stored, such as the bathroom or kitchen, and the use of practical reminders, most often a pillbox. This research was conducted by occupational therapists, a reminder of the importance of working with all disciplines in providing oversight into the care of older adults.

Another creative oversight of patients in the community is faith-based or parish nurses. Twenty faith-based community nurses working with 67 participants at a brown bag medication review event had a positive effect on medication adherence (mean age 75.8 ± 8.9 years).[54] The study did not script the interaction and did not focus on medication adherence, but the intervention does provide nurses with a reminder of creative ways to influence patient behaviors.

IMPLICATIONS FOR PRACTICE

Because adherence is not a one-dimension problem, nurses have a wide variety of interventions available when working with older adults. The nursing process is foundational to helping patients achieve a successful outcome. Nurses must first assess if nonadherence is a concern. Objective measures, such as cholesterol levels or pill counts, may not always be possible. Nurses can readily use the evidence-based Morisky 4-item or 8-item survey[24,25] to screen for nonadherence (see **Box 1**). If a patient is believed nonadherent, the nurse should then explore for intentional and unintentional factors across the 5 dimensions in the WHO model (see **Fig. 1**): social/economic factors, health system–health care team factors, therapy factors, condition factors, and patient factors.[11] Having a problem and a cause (a diagnosis), the nurse can then individualize the plan of care with the patient and the patient's support system (see **Box 2**). Barriers to implementation must be anticipated and the plan adjusted or even changed entirely to effectively arrive at a positive outcome. Thereafter, follow-up is required to evaluate the individual approach. Adherence is again assessed, the patient and significant other's satisfaction with the plan should be assessed, and, if possible, an objective measure should be obtained (pill count and electronic monitoring systems). The mnemonic, SIMPLE, offered by Atreja and colleagues,[55] serves as a basic reminder of the steps needed to enhance patient adherence (**Box 3**).

The issue of medication nonadherence is not new. Research has been ongoing for years. There are, however, increasingly more and more tools to influence patient care. Nurses need to lead the way in researching interventions that can affect medication adherence in older adults, working with the current generation of older adults to develop plans that meet their needs and using interventions that make sense to them. In addition, nurses need to begin now to explore interventions that will work with the rising generation of older adults—those baby boomers who are more comfortable with different skill sets but may have unique barriers to address. Nurses can be integral in designing and testing products that could be valuable with the rising population of older adults, who are more prone to using technology every day. Nurses are cautioned, however, not to abandon practical interventions, because the expense alone of monthly cell phone bills and other technology will limit the availability of these interventions to some older adults. Nurses will be instrumental in laying the ethical foundation for all product designs and research with this growing technology and overriding issues of medication adherence. Nurses can contribute to finding solutions to medication adherence through policy, systems, practice, and research, with the first step being effective communication with older adults and their caregivers.

Box 3
Atreja and Colleagues' SIMPLE mnemonic to guide adherence interventions

S: Simplify regimen.

I: Impart knowledge.

M: Modify patient beliefs and human behavior.

P: Provide communication and trust.

L: Leave the bias.

E: Evaluate adherence.

From Atreja A, Bellam N, Levy SR. Strategies to enhance patient adherence: making it simple. MedGenMed 2005;7(1):4.

REFERENCES

1. Osterberg L, Blaschke T. Adherence to medication. N Engl J Med 2005;353: 487–97.
2. Vincent GK, Velkoff VA. The next four decades. The older population in the United States: 2010 to 2050. In Current Population Reports. 2010. Available at: http://www.census.gov/prod/2010pubs/p25-1138.pdf. Accessed September 19, 2013.
3. Bodenheimer T. Coordinating care–a perilous journey through the health care system. N Engl J Med 2008;358:1064–71. http://dx.doi.org/10.1056/NEJMhpr0706165.
4. Qato DM, Alexander GC, Conti RM, et al. Use of prescription and over-the-counter medications and dietary supplements among older adults in the United States. JAMA 2008;300:2867–78. http://dx.doi.org/10.1001/jama.2008.892.
5. Peterson AM, Takiya L, Finley R. Meta-analysis of trials of interventions to improve medication adherence. Am J Health Syst Pharm 2003;60:657–65.
6. Haynes RB, Ackloo E, Sahota N, et al. Interventions for enhancing medication adherence. Cochrane Database Syst Rev 2008;(2). CD000011. http://dx.doi.org/10.1002/14651858.CD000011.pub3.
7. Viswanathan M, Golin CE, Jones CD, et al. Medication adherence interventions: comparative effectiveness. Closing the quality gap: revisiting the state of the science. Evidence Report No. 208. (Prepared by RTI International–University of North Carolina Evidence-based Practice Center under contract no. 290-2007-10056-I.). AHRQ Publication No. 12–E010-EF. Rockville (MD): Agency for Healthcare Research and Quality September; 2012. Available at: http://www.effectivehealthcare.ahrq.gov/ehc/products/296/1248/EvidenceReport208_CQGMedAdherence_FinalReport_20120905.pdf. Accessed September 19, 2013.
8. Marcum ZA, Gellad WF. Medication adherence to multidrug regimens. Clin Geriatr Med 2012;28:287–300. http://dx.doi.org/10.1016/j.cger.2012.01.008.
9. Topinkova E, Baeyens JP, Michel JP, et al. Evidence-based strategies for the optimization of pharmacotherapy in older people. Drugs Aging 2012;29:477–94.
10. Centers for Disease Control and Prevention (CDC). Medication adherence, CDC's noon conference, March 27, 2013. Centers for Disease Control and Prevention; 2013. Available at: http://www.cdc.gov.proxy.its.virginia.edu/primarycare/materials/medication/. Accessed August 10, 2013.
11. Sabate E. Adherence to long-term therapies: evidence for action. Geneva (Switzerland): World Health Organization; 2003. Available at: http://whqlibdoc.who.int/publications/2003/9241545992.pdf. Accessed September 19, 2013.
12. Ho PM, Bryson CL, Rumsfeld JS. Medication adherence: its importance in cardiovascular outcomes. Circulation 2009;119:3028–35. http://dx.doi.org/10.1161/CIRCULATIONAHA.108.768986.
13. Lehane E, McCarthy G. Intentional and unintentional medication non-adherence: a comprehensive framework for clinical research and practice? A discussion paper. Int J Nurs Stud 2007;44:1468–77.
14. Nazareth I, Burton A, Shulman S, et al. A pharmacy discharge plan for hospitalized elderly patients–a randomized controlled trial. Age Ageing 2001;30(1): 33–40.
15. Volume CI, Farris KB, Kassam R, et al. Pharmaceutical care research and education project: patient outcomes. J Am Pharm Assoc (Wash) 2001;41:411–20.
16. Ruppar TM, Conn VS, Russell CL. Medication adherence interventions for older adults: literature review. Res Theory Nurs Pract 2008;22(2):114–47.

17. Conn VS, Hafdahl AR, Cooper PS, et al. Interventions to improve medication adherence among older adults: meta-analysis of adherence outcomes among randomized controlled trials. Gerontologist 2009;49:447–62. http://dx.doi.org/10.1093/geront/gnp037.

18. Banning M. A review of interventions used to improve adherence to medication in older people. Int J Nurs Stud 2009;46:1505–15. http://dx.doi.org/10.1016/j.ijnurstu.2009.03.011.

19. Russell CL, Ruppar TM, Matteson M. Improving medication adherence: moving from intention and motivation to a personal systems approach. Nurs Clin North Am 2011;46(3):271–81. http://dx.doi.org/10.1016/j.cnur.2011.05.004.

20. Bandura A. Health promotion from the perspective of social cognitive theory. In: Norman P, Abraham C, Conner M, editors. Understanding and changing health behavior: from health beliefs to self-regulation. Amsterdam: Harwood Academic Publishers; 2000. p. 299–339.

21. Ajzen I, Fishbein M. Understanding attitudes and predicting social behavior. Englewood Cliffs (NJ): Prentice-Hall; 1980.

22. Leventhal H, Nerenz DR, Straus A. Self-regulation and the mechanisms for symptom appraisal. In: Mechanic D, editor. Symptoms, illness behavior, and help-seeking. New York: Prodist; 1982. p. 55–86.

23. Alemi F, Neuhauser D, Ardito S, et al. Continuous self-improvement: systems thinking in a personal context. Jt Comm J Qual Improv 2000;26(2):74–86.

24. Morisky DE, Green LW, Levine DM. Concurrent and predictive validity of a self-reported measure of medication adherence. Med Care 1986;24(1):67–74.

25. Lavsa SM, Holzworth A, Ansani NT. Selection of a validated scale for measuring medication adherence. J Am Pharm Assoc (2003) 2011;51(1):90–4. http://dx.doi.org/10.1331/JAPhA.2011.09154.

26. Sirey JA, Greenfield A, Weinberger MI, et al. Medication beliefs and self-reported adherence among community-dwelling older adults. Clin Ther 2013;35(2):153–60.

27. Unni EJ, Farris KB. Unintentional non-adherence and belief in medicines in older adults. Patient Educ Couns 2011;83(2):265–8. http://dx.doi.org/10.1016/j.pec.2010.05.006.

28. Shi L, Liu J, Fonseca V, et al. Correlation between adherence rates measured by MEMS and self-reported questionnaires: a meta-analysis. Health Qual Life Outcomes 2010;99:8. http://dx.doi.org/10.1186/1477-7525-8-99.

29. MeadWestvaco. MEMSCap Medication Event Monitoring System. 2013. Available at: http://www.mwvaardex.com/Products/DataCollection/MEMSCap/index.htm. Accessed September 19, 2013.

30. Demonceau J, Ruppar T, Kristanto P, et al. Identification and assessment of adherence-enhancing interventions in studies assessing medication adherence through electronically compiled drug dosing histories: a systematic literature review and meta-analysis. Drugs 2013;73:545–62.

31. ePill. E-pill medication reminders: pill dispenser, vibrating watch, pill box timer, alarms. Available at: http://www.epill.com/. Accessed September 19, 2013.

32. Joe J, Demiris G. Older adults and mobile phones for health: a review. J Biomed Inform 2013;46:947–54. http://dx.doi.org/10.1016/j.jbi.2013.06.008.

33. Fenerty SD, West C, Davis SA, et al. The effect of reminder systems on patients' adherence to treatment. Patient Prefer Adherence 2012;6:127–35. http://dx.doi.org/10.2147/PPA.S26314.

34. Vervloet M, Linn AJ, van Weert JC, et al. The effectiveness of interventions using electronic reminders to improve adherence to chronic medication: a systematic review of the literature. J Am Med Inform Assoc 2012;19:696–704. http://dx.doi.org/10.1136/amiajnl-2011-000748.

35. Smith A. Smartphone ownership–2013 update. Pew Research Center. 2013. Available at: http://www.pewinternet.org/~/media/Files/Reports/2013/PIP_Smartphone_adoption_2013.pdf. Accessed September 19, 2013.

36. Miller JT. Simpliifed smartphones for boomers and seniors. In The Huffington Post. 2013. Available at: http://www.huffingtonpost.com/jim-t-miller/smart phones-for-seniors_b_2843091.html. Accessed September 19, 2013.

37. Dayer L, Heldenbrand S, Anderson P, et al. Smartphone medication adherence apps: potential benefits to patients and providers. J Am Pharm Assoc (2003) 2013;53(2):172–81. http://dx.doi.org/10.1331/JAPhA.2013.12202.

38. Heinrich C, Kuiper RA. Using handheld devices to promote medication adherence in chronic illness. J Nurse Pract 2012;8(4):288.

39. GreatCall. GreatCall - Official home of Jitterbug, 5Star, Medical apps. Available at: http://www.greatcall.com/. Accessed September 19, 2013.

40. Samsung. Galaxy S4-tips and tricks, Samsung mobile article. Available at: http://www.samsung.com/us/article/tips-tricks-galaxy-s-4. Accessed September 19, 2013.

41. Zickuhr K. Tablet ownership 2013. Pew Research Center. 2013. Available at: http://pewinternet.org/Reports/2013/Tablet-Ownership-2013.aspx. Accessed September 19, 2013.

42. Claris Companion. Communication for seniors-Claris Companion. Available at: http://www.clariscompanion.com/. Accessed September 19, 2013.

43. Boulos MN, Wheeler S, Tavares C, et al. How smartphones are changing the face of mobile and participatory healthcare: an overview, with example from eCAALYX. Biomed Eng Online 2011;10:24. http://dx.doi.org/10.1186/1475-925X-10-24.

44. Epstein RS. Medication adherence: hope for improvement? Mayo Clin Proc 2011;86:268–70. http://dx.doi.org/10.4065/mcp.2011.0123.

45. American Heart Association (AHA) First Consulting Group. When I'm 64: how boomers will change health care. Chicago: American Hospital Association; 2007.

46. Brandt NJ, Hanna K, Walters S. Medication management and older adults. J Gerontol Nurs 2013;39(2):3–7.

47. Marrufo G, Dixit A, Perlroth D, et al. Medication Therapy Management in a chronically ill population: interim report. Acumen, LLC. Centers for Medicare and Medicaid Services. 2013. Available at: http://innovation.cms.gov/Files/reports/MTM-Interim-Report-01-2013.pdf. Accessed September 19, 2013.

48. U.S. Department of Health and Human Services. Affordable Care Act. Available at: http://www.hhs.gov/opa/affordable-care-act/index.html. Accessed September 19, 2013.

49. Kux L. "Script your future" medication adherence campaign. Docket No. FDA–2013–N–0012. Food and Drug Administration. 2013. Available at: https://www.federalregister.gov/articles/2013/06/06/2013-13447/script-your-future-medication-adherence-campaign. Accessed September 19, 2013.

50. Honigberg R, Gordon M, Wisniewski AC. Supporting patient medication adherence: ensuring coordination, quality and outcomes (White Paper). 2011. Available at: http://adhereforhealth.org/wp-content/uploads/pdf/URAC-MedAdherence_WP.pdf. Accessed March 11, 2014.

51. Ownby RL, Hertzog C, Czaja SJ. Tailored information and automated reminding to improve medication adherence in Spanish- and English-speaking elders treated for memory impairment. Clin Gerontol 2012;35:221–38.

52. Campbell NL, Boustani MA, Skopelja EN, et al. Medication adherence in older adults with cognitive impairment: a systematic evidence-based review. Am J Geriatr Pharmacother 2012;10(3):165–77. http://dx.doi.org/10.1016/j.amjopharm.2012.04.004.

53. Sanders MJ, Van Oss T. Using daily routines to promote medication adherence in older adults. Am J Occup Ther 2013;67(1):91–9. http://dx.doi.org/10.5014/ajot.2013.005033.

54. Shillam CR, Orton VJ, Waring D, et al. Faith community nurses & brown bag events help older adults manage meds. J Christ Nurs 2013;30(2):90–6.

55. Atreja A, Bellam N, Levy SR. Strategies to enhance patient adherence: making it simple. MedGenMed 2005;7(1):4.

Keeping Older Adults Safe, Protected, and Healthy by Preventing Financial Exploitation

Janet Sullivan-Wilson, PhD, RN[a],*,
Kimethria L. Jackson, RN, MSN, FNP, APRN[b]

KEYWORDS

- Financial • Exploitation • Older adults • Elderly • Abuse

KEY POINTS

- Financial or material exploitation is one of the most prevalent types of older adult maltreatments.
- An older adult's health is a risk factor for financial exploitation and at risk when financially exploited.
- The impact of financial exploitation on older adults is greater than other age groups because the loss of irreplaceable assets, savings, and resources can compromise independence, security, and psychological well-being, leading to depression, suicide, hopelessness, confusion, and premature death.
- Risk factors include minority status (especially African American), women, age in the late 70s and older, and diminishing cognitive capacity.
- In most states, nurses and other health care professionals are mandated reporters to Adult Protective Service for suspected financial exploitation.

INTRODUCTION

I had an aneurysm and they think I don't know what's going on around me, and they assume that I don't know anything, and they took advantage of me, each one of them. What helped me is when I really started coming out of my aneurysm

Funding Sources: Donald W. Reynolds Center of Geriatric Nursing Excellence, The Substance Abuse and Mental Health Services Administration and the American Nurse Association Minority Fellowship Program.

Conflict of Interest: None.

[a] Donald W. Reynolds Center of Geriatric Nursing Excellence Community Based Interdisciplinary Research, College of Nursing, University of Oklahoma Health Sciences Center, 1100 North Stonewall, Room 363, PO Box 26901, Oklahoma City, OK 73126-0901, USA; [b] Donald W. Reynolds Center of Geriatric Nursing Excellence, College of Nursing, University of Oklahoma Health Sciences Center, 1100 North Stonewall, PO Box 26901, Oklahoma City, OK 73126-0901, USA

* Corresponding author.

E-mail address: janet-wilson@ouhsc.edu

*and I started looking at things and putting two and two together. They find some-
body that's in a state like I was with a brain aneurysm and they know they got
money coming in and if they don't have an overseer of that person, they get
used, especially from family members. They stole from a disabled man, knowing
he had brain problems, knowing what he was taking money for, knowing all this.*
—Quote from an 82-year-old man recovering from a brain aneurysm talking
with the authors about his family taking his money from him.

Financial or material exploitation as described above is one of the 7 types of elder maltreatments defined by the National Center on Elder Abuse as, "...the illegal or
improper use of an elder's funds, property, or assets. Examples include, but are not
limited to, cashing an elderly person's checks without authorization or permission;
forging an older person's signature; misusing or stealing an older person's money
or possessions; coercing or deceiving an older person into signing any document
(eg, contracts or will); and the improper use of conservatorship, guardianship, or power of attorney."[1]

Financial exploitation (FE) is now thought to be one of the most prevalent,[2–5] yet
least detected and reported types of older adult maltreatments, that include physical,
emotional, and sexual maltreatment; neglect; self-neglect; and abandonment.[6] FE of
older adults by family members, caregivers, stranger scams, and Medicare fraud
causes an estimated $2.9 billion loss per year for the victims, thus depriving them
of needed resources as they age, need more health care services, and experience
chronic illness.[7] Because adults over the age of 65 become 20% of the population
by 2030, the incidence of FE is only expected to escalate.[4]

"When older adults lose their income and resources through financial exploitation
they feel trapped, confused, and abused," testified Mickey Rooney before
Congress in 2011.[8] Without income and resources, FE victims have fewer health
care options and are at a higher risk for poor health outcomes, such as depression, chronic illnesses, substance abuse, and premature death (**Box 1** for FE
signs).[9,10]

FE may occur in isolation (pure FE) or co-occur with physical/sexual abuse and
neglect (hybrid FE). Pure FE and hybrid FE are experienced differently by older
adults in that pure FE offenders are usually not related to the older adult, much
like a white collar crime. Hybrid FE often has more adverse events for the older adult,
as in family domestic violence, where there is a long-standing relationship between
the victim and the perpetrator with more frequent and lengthier occurrences.[11] The
importance of distinguishing between these 2 forms of FE is that each may require
different assessments, interventions, and management from health care, legal,
and social service providers, although this still has to be empirically tested.[11]
However, if FE by its very nature involves some form of (albeit subtle) deceit, coercion, or undue influence (ie, a form of emotional maltreatment) on the part of the
offender as research evidence suggests, this causes all forms of FE to be hybrid
by definition.

Another perspective is that the co-occurrence of FE with emotional and coercive
tactics of manipulation, deceit, and threats[12] is an eroding and dehumanizing process
that over time is a catalyst for offenders to escalate to neglect and physical and sexual maltreatment.[7] Research evidence as well as anecdotal accounts of FE indeed
point to the interrelationships of FE, physical, sexual maltreatment, and neglect
occurring together.[7] However, more study is needed to explore and validate these interrelationships. Nurses, doctors, and social service providers must first be aware of
FE to be able to detect, report, and document FE to keep older adults safe, protected,
and healthy.

Box 1
Signs of FE

The National Center on Elder Abuse Signs of Financial Exploitation of an Older Adult

- Sudden changes in bank account or banking practice, including an unexplained withdrawal of large sums of money by a person accompanying the elder;

- The inclusion of additional names on an elder's bank signature card;

- Unauthorized withdrawal of the elder's funds using the elder's automated teller machine card;

- Abrupt changes in a will or other financial documents;

- Unexplained disappearance of funds or valuable possessions;

- Substandard care being provided or bills unpaid despite the availability of adequate financial resources;

- Discovery of an elder's signature being forged for financial transactions or for the titles of his/her possessions;

- Sudden appearance of previously uninvolved relatives claiming their rights to an elder's affairs and possessions;

- Unexplained sudden transfer of assets to a family member or someone outside the family;

- The provision of services that are not necessary; and

- An elder's report of FE.

From US Department of Health and Human Services Administration on Aging. National Center on Elder Abuse. Available at: http://ncea.aoa.gov/FAQ/Type_Abuse/#financial. Accessed March 13, 2014.

FE AS AN OLDER ADULT HEALTH PROBLEM

FE is a health care problem for 5 reasons[4]: (1) FE victims are health care clients who are in need of specific types of care; (2) FE offenders are health caregivers and employees who are in positions of trust with victims who depend on them and need their care; (3) older adult health problems arise as a result of FE; (4) FE victimization often occurs within the health care context and/or setting; (5) the risks for FE are tied to the health of older adults.

FE Victims Are Health Care Clients in Need of Specific Types of Care

As some people age, physical and/or cognitive health diminishes to the point where they need to rely on other people for both physical and fiscal help. The assistance needed may range from help with paying the bills or buying groceries to granting a legal, written power of attorney (POA) to a trusted person to act on their behalf in all financial and some health care matters. Depending on the level of care needed by an older adult, there are risks for FE happening. For example, when a caregiver pockets the change after buying groceries, this is FE. Gaining access to automated teller machine cards, credit cards, savings/checking accounts, and investment funds to withdraw funds for personal use, such as buying and selling services and goods, happens with misuse of POAs.[13] The more assets a dependent, frail, and aged older adult has, the more vulnerable she or he will be to more extensive forms of FE, such as misuse of POAs.[11,13]

Although FE can occur alone, it is not unusual for an older adult to be financially exploited, neglected, and physically maltreated at the same time,[5] so nurses must look for occurrences of more than one type of abuse when assessing for FE. If further investigation reveals that FE is indeed a gateway to other cooccurring abuses,[7] this supports the argument that early FE assessment and reporting is a prevention strategy for other forms of elder maltreatment.

Health Caregivers and Employees as FE Offenders

Primary contact offenders or people with close relationships with the older adults (children, caregivers, relatives) are the majority of the FE offenders,[5] who exploit by direct theft; by coercing property transfers in exchange for better care; by improper use of POA, joint signatures, or joint tenancies to gain assets; and by conversion of public benefits or entitlement checks for services not covered. Secondary contacts (generally nonrelatives) financially exploit with home repair, insurance, and medical frauds; confidence games; and telemarketing scams.[14] In a case-controlled study of 370 older adults referred to Protective Services for Older Adults, Erie County, New York, almost 40% of the perpetrators in this sample were nonrelative perpetrators that included home health aides, other paid or nonpaid caregivers, neighbors, people living in the home, and strangers.[5]

What is clear from the myriad ways older adults are financially exploited is that this population is targeted for FE because of their vulnerabilities of advancing age, assets, declining health, and cognitive capacity. The following still-unsolved criminal case is from the Federal Bureau of Investigation's Wanted List and is prototypic of FE by a trusted nonrelative caregiver:

> Monica Michelle Brown is wanted for her alleged involvement in a scheme that defrauded an elderly man of over $250,000. In July of 2011, a financial institution contacted the FBI in Oklahoma City, Oklahoma, regarding the financial exploitation of a 97-year-old man residing in an Oklahoma City nursing home. In December 2010, someone set up online banking on the victim's bank account without his permission. Shortly thereafter, checks were initiated through the online system and were sent to various people, including Brown. Subsequent investigation discovered Brown and an accomplice had been employed at the nursing home and were responsible for financially exploiting the elderly man.

> On November 7, 2012, Brown was indicted by a federal grand jury in the United States District Court for the Western District of Oklahoma with one count of conspiracy, two counts of mail fraud, and five counts of forged securities. A federal arrest warrant was issued for Brown's arrest on November 8, 2012, also in the United States District Court, Western District of Oklahoma. Brown was also charged with four counts of writing bogus checks by the Cleveland County, Oklahoma, District Attorney. Brown may be residing with family in Arkansas.[15]

This case illustrates some of the unique (and therefore the serious) characteristics of FE perpetration: FE is premeditated, takes place within the context of a health care relationship, uses different means to steal assets, is "entrenched" (long duration) and "intractable" (mutual dependency of the older adult and the perpetrator),[13] and lacks witnesses who may detect and report the criminal maltreatment.

Health Problems Arise as a Result of FE

Medications, appointments to primary care practitioners and/or specialists, pre-ventative screenings and checkups, medical treatments, and rehabilitation are a few of the health care services that are neglected when older adults are deprived of assets and resources that they have saved for their long-term care. As a result, mounting evidence suggests that because of the deprivation of health services that FE causes, poor health,[16] confusion, dementia,[17] behavioral problems,[18] depression,[14,19] dislocation from homes, and premature mortality[7,8] are associated with FE.

FE Victimization Often Occurs Within the Health Care Context or Setting

FE may take place in a health care physical setting, such as the home, community cen-ter, hospital, clinic, day care, respite center, long-term care facility, and so on. How-ever, a preponderance of FE occurs more within the health care context, despite the setting. In other words, older adults who need more health services because of increasing physical/emotional dependency and diminishing cognitive capacity and who put a great deal of trust in another person for their care are more vulnerable to FE victimization. Susceptible victims can be older adults who are almost completely dependent on others (financial prisoners), those who have lost interest in taking care of their finances (slipping), and grieving widows who welcome exploiters taking over fiscal tasks they do not enjoy or comprehend.[4]

FE Risks Are Tied to Older Adult Health

Although not all older adults are vulnerable, aging increases certain vulnerabilities that increase risks for FE from primary and secondary contacts. Primary contacts, such as children, spouses, family members, or friends, are those people who have a relation-ship with the older adult. Secondary contacts are nonrelatives who either target older adults or through greed gain access to their financial assets and resources through medical, financial, insurance, home repair, telemarketing, Internet, or confidence schemes.[14] Older adults are at risk for a wide range of FEs through both their primary and their secondary contacts.

Risks vary among the different types of older adult maltreatments, but an elder's age, frailty, and dependency are significant predictors of any type of maltreatment. Older age (late 70s and older), living alone, home ownership, lack of financial knowledge, and/or cognitive deficits (that become apparent when problems appear in mismanaging finances) are all associated with increased risk for being exploited financially.[5] Female gender, social network size, severity of the physical and/or emotional disability or illness, and ethnicity (especially African Americans) have also been implicated in increasing an older adult's vulnerability to FE.[5,12,16–18,20,21]

FE OF MINORITIES: AFRICAN AMERICAN ELDERS

Understanding of FE in minority groups is limited with FE of African American Elder (AAE) studies having the largest but limited number. African Americans made up 8.3% of the older adult population in 2008 and, by the year 2050, African Americans will account for 11% of the elder population.[19] FE has an impact on the health out-comes and quality of life of AAEs, an expanding, vulnerable group with high rates of health disparities and mortality due to chronic health conditions.[5] The loss of financial resources reduces available health care options for needed care and services and further engenders health disparities for AAEs. This loss places AAEs in double jeopardy for adverse health outcomes. FE of AAEs can result in loss of human rights, human dignity, and human life.[7]

Prevalence rates for elder abuse FE are thought to be higher among AAEs as compared with non-African Americans[12,22] and rank first among the types of abuse most commonly reported by AAEs.[23] AAEs are also more likely than their Caucasian counterparts to report FE.[24] Multigenerational living arrangements, unique to the African American culture, are possible covariates to FE,[12] with an offspring of the elder most often the offender.[24]

Another inquiry, although acknowledging scarce literature related to FE among AAEs and limitations in study sample size, found that both AAEs and non-African Americans had equally high rates of FE as compared with other forms of abuse, thus refuting other findings.[25] Because of the small number of studies, small sample sizes, and differences among findings, FE in AAEs is a serious minority concern that deserves more investigation.

Gender differences among victims in AAEs showed that there was no significant difference in the experience of FE between AAEs male and female victims, although the potential for abuse was greater for AAE men who lived with spouses and children than AAE women who lived alone or with children.[26] Most of the perpetrators of AAEs tended to be female daughters not living with their elder parent who were not financially dependent on the elder, or a substance abuser. Half of the female perpetrators had a legal financial responsibility to the elder, although equal numbers of men and women were informal caregivers.[26] This finding contradicts the stereotype of AAE perpetrators being male substance abusers who are dependents of the AAEs and supports the hypothesis that perpetrators may be responding to other life issues that are not related to caregiver stress or financial dependence on the elder.[22]

AAEs are already a vulnerable population with health disparities and high rates of mortality. FE of AAEs leaves this group in a dilemma. There are differences between what the majority culture deems FE and what AAEs and the African American culture experience as FE. Although evidence suggests the prevalence of FE in AAEs is increasing, the understanding is limited, in part due to small nonrepresentative samples in few empiric and qualitative studies. Although inclusion of AAEs in studies with larger sample sizes has improved, the number of studies focusing exclusively on AAEs experiencing FE remains sparse. FE must be studied more fully in various ethnic groups to understand FE fully. The social context, cultural norms, values, and beliefs in which FE occurs for AAEs are different from other cultures. Differences influence the perception of FE, reporting, responding, and help seeking of FE in AAEs as well as first responders. The discrepancy should be eliminated by further exploration of FE to develop appropriate treatment and effective interventions that will prevent the abusive crime of FE in AAEs.

UNDERDETECTING AND UNDERREPORTING FE

Only a small percentage of elder abuse is ever reported and FE is less likely than other forms of maltreatments to be detected or reported.[27,28] Most nurses and physicians underestimate the prevalence of elder abuse in general and do not think detecting and reporting FE is their responsibility, even though it is one of the most prevalent of the elder maltreatments that devastates older adults and families.[28] To be sure, there are many reasons nurses and other health care practitioners do not detect FE and therefore do not report it as maltreatment. An overriding explanation is that FE continues to be hidden from society.[29] Ageism and entitlement (eg, to inheritances and personal property of aging parents) prevail today. "Why spend so much of our inheritance on Mom's care?," is not an unheard question in the health care setting, belying the fact that it is embezzlement to deprive an older adult of their funds needed for their care.

A more pragmatic explanation of why FE goes undetected and underreported is that detecting is difficult when there is a lack of knowledge, understanding, and training about FE signs/symptoms, screening tools, and reporting steps in nursing and medical curriculums today.[21,30,31] Along with this elder maltreatment, science is not yet advanced enough to have validated strategies (protocols) that give guidance to collaboratively manage FE in the clinical arena.[21,32] Lack of time and reimbursement mechanisms for FE elder abuse assessments discourage implementation of assessment intervention protocols for FE.[21] The fear and discomfort in handling the ethical, legal matters of abuse within the context of the therapeutic relationship[21,30,33] cause health care providers to withdraw from taking action when FE is suspected.

Older adults' shame, embarrassment, and fear of the potential harmful consequences of perpetrator retaliation when reporting FE[32] interact with health care practitioner anxieties to form a type of mutual withdrawal when dealing with FE. FE perpetrators play into this by threats, intimidation, deceit, and lying to get what they want from the older adult. Our fragmented systems of health care, law enforcement, and social services are often uncommunicative with one another when FE cases are discovered, thus leaving practitioners without the benefit of a collaborative response to help one another manage the safety and protection of older adults.[29] These difficulties in detecting, reporting, and managing FE of older adults are formidable, but the interdisciplinary fields of child abuse and intimate partner violence have had similar problems in detection and reporting that have been resolved by academics and practitioners partnering to advance the science to make changes.

FE PREVENTION INTERVENTION STRATEGIES

Detecting and reporting are still thought to be the most beneficial interventions for any type of elder maltreatment, including FE.[10] Not only are health care practitioners legally mandated to report FE, but by so doing this action has the potential to trigger a system of collaborative community resources and responses to investigate, provide assistance and safety, and connect older adult victims with social services and interventions.

Several elder maltreatment assessment tools have been developed to aid in detecting and reporting FE and elder maltreatment.[34-37] These instruments provide the structure and documentation necessary for older adult care, protection, and safety care planning. Most of these instruments focus on all the elder maltreatments and have a few questions related to FE. Practitioners can choose an assessment form that meets their needs and develop procedures and protocols that give guidelines specific to their agency (**Table 1** lists FE assessment tools).

The 82-item self-report Older Adult Financial Exploitation Measure, specific to FE, shows the most promise for accurate FE detection and subsequent responding/reporting by clinical practitioners.[36] The 82 questions were developed from an FE conceptual framework the researchers developed that identified 6 clusters of FE in descending severity: theft and scams; financial victimization; financial entitlement; coercion; signs of possible FE; money management.[38] This instrument can be

Table 1
FE assessment tools

Name of Instrument	Domain/Concept	Validity and Reliability
Older Adult Financial Exploitation Measure (OAFEM)[36]	FE	Discriminant validity-unidimensional 79-item variance explained 44.3% residual 7.0%, 54 item (42.3%, 7.7%), 30 item (45.2%, 10%); interrater reliability demonstrated for 79-item scale; internal consistency: 79-item person reliability 0.92 (corresponds to $\alpha = 0.96$) item reliability 0.95; 54-item person reliability 0.88 ($\alpha = 0.95$) item reliability 0.95; 30-item person reliability 0.85 ($\alpha = 0.93$) item reliability 0.96
Elder Assessment Instrument (EAI)[34]	Physical, sexual abuse, neglect, exploitation, and abandonment	Internal consistency reliability ($\alpha = 0.84$); test/retest reliability = 0.83 ($P<.0001$)
Single Page Elder Abuse Assessment and Management Tool[37]	Physical, sexual abuse, neglect, exploitation, and abandonment	Not reported
EIFEE Clinician FE Scale: http://www.nasaa. org/1733/eiffe/	FE	Not reported

reduced with permission of the researchers to a user-friendly 25-item version of the tool that is more manageable in health care settings.

Daly[39] recommends using not only well-established EM assessment tools to identify risks and plan care and safety/security measures for older adult maltreatment but also an interdisciplinary team approach to detect and report elder maltreatment. Fiduciary Abuse Specialist Teams have been established throughout the country and comprise both public and private interprofessionals representing Adult Protective Services, law enforcement, prosecution, guardians, Long Term Care Ombudsman, banking, health care, real estate, and so on. Teams may meet monthly to review one to 3 complex FE cases.[40] There is no research, however, to test if these teams have reduced the rate of FE or increased FE detection and reporting.

Other programs and interventions have been developed to increase FE detection and reporting,[24] but these programs do not use validated FE assessment tools or protocols and there is no evaluation as to whether health care FE detection and reporting rates increase as a result of their assessments (**Table 2**). Presently there are tools to determine diminished financial capacity in older adults with cognitive impairments, indicating a potential risk for FE, but these studies do not assess if FE has occurred as a result.[31] There are educational strategies to improve health care practitioners' knowledge and attitudes about elder abuse[12,32,33] but these do not test how that knowledge affects practitioners' FE management, detection, and reporting rates. A next step in elder abuse science is to test interventions that use a systematic and collaborative assessment intervention protocol that addresses the difficulties practitioners are having with detecting and reporting FE.

Table 2
Older adult FE prevention programs

Financial Exploitation Prevention Programs for Older Adults	Program Description/Resources
Consumer Financial Protection Bureau	Consumer information regarding FE and new financial resource tool, *Money Smart for Older Adults*, to help older adults and their caregivers prevent elder FE across the country: http://www.consumerfinance.gov/pressreleases/fdic-and-cfpb-collaborate-to-develop-a-tool-for-older-adults-to-prevent-financial-exploitation/
Elder Investment Fraud and Financial Exploitation (EIFFE) Prevention Program	A national collaborative program of state securities regulators, Investor Protection Trust, National Adult Protective Services Association (NAPSA), American Academy of Family Physicians, National Area Health Education Center Organization, and National Association of Geriatric Education Centers, to educate medical professionals, caregivers about how to identify older adults vulnerable to financial abuse. A video, clinician's pocket guide, patient information brochure, and a brochure regarding the ABC's of reporting FE are available free on this Web site. 28 states are participating in this education program: http://www.nasaa.org/1733/eiffe/
Florida Department of Elder Affairs	http://elderaffairs.state.fl.us/doea/elderabuseprevention/Financial%20Exploitation_English_web.pdf
Financial Abuse Specialist Teams (FAST)	The National Center on Elder Abuse gives resources and information about how to develop collaborative FE prevention programs: http://ncea.aoa.gov/Stop_Abuse/Teams/FAST/. The Los Angeles County Fiduciary Abuse Specialist Team was one of the first FAST teams in the country.[40]
New York State Office for the Aging	US Administration for Community Living (ACL) 3-y grant to pilot an enhanced multidisciplinary team with a forensic accountant as part of the team to investigate FE of older adults: http://www.aging.ny.gov/News/2012/2012PR04.cfm
Coalition Against Financial Exploitation of the Elderly (CAFEE)	County level collaborative that functions similar to an FAST: http://www.okdhs.org/NR/rdonlyres/767B1946-A9C8-44A7-988C-1867697B4A57/0/0820_CAFEE_ASD_05012008.pdf
Oregon Senior Financial Abuse Coalition	Statewide program, Preventing and Responding to Senior Financial Abuse in Oregon: http://www.oregon.gov/dhs/spd/pubs/finabuse_eng.pdf
Organizations to Protect Older Adults	National Adult Protective Services Association: http://www.napsa-now.org/ National Center on Elder Abuse: http://www.ncea.aoa.gov/ National Committee for the Prevention of Elder Abuse: http://www.preventelderabuse.org/

SUMMARY

FE is an older adult health problem that has gone unrecognized and untreated far too long by health care practitioners and academics. Lack of awareness that FE is an older adult maltreatment causes older adults devastating losses, unnecessary health problems, and premature mortality. If FE is as prevalent as research suggests, then clinical practitioners and academics must partner to provide health care clinicians with the knowledge, skills, and tools necessary to detect, respond, and manage the safety and care of older adults.[4] Nurses and other health care professionals are in a unique position of being first responders to FE. Nurses are usually the first to see and know when maltreatment occurs. Because nurses are mandated reporters of elder maltreatment in most states in the country, best evidence thus far supports *assessing* for FE and needed health care services that result from FE with the interdisciplinary community team; *reporting* to Adult Protective Services; *documenting* the care, safety, and protection of identified older adult FE victims; and *enlisting, referring* to nontraditional resources like domestic violence services to help with short-term and long-term safety planning. Recent evidence indicates that FE victim health care intervention may vary according to needs, ethnicity, and gender. Interventions such as case management, hospitalization, emergency department treatment, home care, out-patient treatment, and referral to social, domestic violence, and legal services are some of the strategies that an interdisciplinary community-based team might consider in the implementation of a care and safety plan.

On a systems level, nursing associations like the American Nurses Association are positioned to provide professional guidelines and expectations (similar to the Intimate Partner Violence Guidelines) for detecting, reporting, and documenting older adult maltreatments that would include FE.

In 2011, FE was labeled as the "crime of the 21st Century."[7] Older Americans today possess 70% of all funds deposited in financial institutions, thus making a large portion of the wealth in the United States controlled by persons age 65 and older.[13] A changing US economy, increased reliance on technology, and growth in the diversity and numbers of aging adults with chronic health conditions suggest that FE will not go away, but will increase in prevalence and novel ways exploiters devise to fiscally take advantage of vulnerable older adults.[14] To be ready for these changes, nurses and the health care industry must become wiser and more efficient in detecting, responding, and reporting FE for the health and welfare of our country's aging adults.

REFERENCES

1. National Center on Elder Abuse. Types of abuse, definition. 2012. Available at: http://ncea.aoa.gov/FAQ/Type_Abuse/. Accessed October 29, 2013.
2. Lachs M, Berman J. Under the radar: New York state elder abuse prevalence study. Weil Cornell Medical Center of Cornell University & New York City Department of the Aging; 2011. Available at: http://www.ocfs.state.ny.us/main/reports/Under%20the%20Radar%2005%2012%2011%20final%20report.pdf. Accessed March 13, 2014.
3. Acierno R, Hernandez MA, Amstadter AB, et al. Prevalence and correlates of emotional, physical, sexual, and financial abuse and potential neglect in the United States: the National Elder Mistreatment Study. Am J Publ Health 2010; 100(2):292–7.
4. Payne BK, Strasser SM. Financial exploitation of older persons in adult care settings: comparisons to physical abuse and the justice system's response. J Elder Abuse Negl 2012;24(3):231–50.
5. Choi NG, Mayer J. Elder abuse, neglect, and exploitation: Risk factors and prevention strategies. J Gerontol Soc Work 2000;33(2):5–25.
6. Yaffe MJ. Detection and reporting of elder abuse. Fam Med 2010;42(2):83.
7. MetLife. The MetLife study of elder financial abuse: crimes of occasion, desperation, and predation against America's Elders, Mature Market Institute. 2011. p. 1–25. Available at: http://www.metlife.com/mmi/research/elder-financial-abuse.html#key. Accessed October 26, 2013.

8. Fox Z. Mickey Rooney testifies before congress on elder abuse, urges others to speak out. Time NewsFeed March 3, 2011. Available at: http://newsfeed.time.com/2011/2003/2003/mickey-rooney-testifies-before-congress-on-elder-abuse-urges-others-to-speak-out/. Accessed August 23, 2013.

9. Wagenaar DB, Rosenbaum R, Page C, et al. Primary care physicians and elder abuse: current attitudes and practices. J Am Osteopath Assoc 2010;110(12):703–11.

10. Lachs MS, Williams CS, O'Brien S, et al. The mortality of elder mistreatment. JAMA 1998;280(5):428–32.

11. Jackson SL, Hafemeister TL. Pure financial exploitation vs. hybrid financial exploitation co-occurring with physical abuse and/or neglect of elderly persons. Psychol Violence 2012;2(3):285–96.

12. Beach SR, Schulz R, Castle NG, et al. Financial exploitation and psychological mistreatment among older adults: differences between African Americans and non-African Americans in a population-based survey. Gerontologist 2010;50(6):744–57.

13. Jackson SL, Hafemeister TL. Financial abuse of elderly people vs. other forms of elder abuse: assessing their dynamics, risk factors, and Society's Response U.S. Department of Justice. Department of Justice Report; 2011. Available at: https://www.ncjrs.gov/pdffiles1/nij/grants/233613.pdf. Accessed March 13, 2014.

14. Payne BK. Crime and elder abuse: an integrated perspective. Springfield (IL): Charles C. Thomas; 2005.

15. FBI. Wanted by the FBI, Federal Bureau of Investigation. 2013. Available at: http://www.fbi.gov/oklahomacity/press-releases/2013/former-employee-of-assisted-living-center-sentenced-to-37-months-in-prison-for-fraud. Accessed March 13, 2014.

16. Pinsker DM, McFarland K. Exploitation in older adults: personal competence correlates of social vulnerability. Neuropsychol Dev Cogn B Aging Neuropsychol Cogn 2010;17(6):673–708.

17. Stamatel JP, Mastrocinque JM. Using National Incident-Based Reporting System (NIBRS) data to understand financial exploitation of the elderly: a research note. Vict Offender 2011;6(2):117–36.

18. Tueth MJ. Exposing financial exploitation of impaired elderly persons. Am J Geriatr Psychiatry 2000;8(2):104–11.

19. Administration on Aging. A statistical profile of black older Americans Aged 65+. 2009. Available at: http://www.aoa.gov/AoARoot/Aging_Statistics/minority_aging/Facts-on-Black-Elderly2009-plain_format.aspx. Accessed October 29, 2013.

20. Lichtenberg PA, Stickney L, Paulson D. Is psychological vulnerability related to the experience of fraud in older adults? Clin Gerontol 2013;36(2):132–46.

21. Halphen JM, Varas GM, Sadowsky JM. Recognizing and reporting elder abuse and neglect. Geriatrics 2009;64(7):13–8.

22. Griffin LW. Elder mistreatment among rural African-Americans. J Elder Abuse Negl 1994;6(1):1–28.

23. Tatara T. Understanding elder abuse in minority populations. Philadelphia: Brunner/Mazel; 1999. p. 13–64.

24. Laumann EO, Leitsch SA, Waite LJ. Elder mistreatment in the United States: prevalence estimates from a nationally representative study. J Gerontol B Psychol Sci Soc Sci 2008;63(4):S248–54.

25. Dimah KP. Patterns of elder abuse and neglect in an Illinois elder abuse and neglect provider agency: a comparative analysis. J Elder Abuse Negl 2001;13(1):27–44.

26. Dimah A, Patricia Dimah K. Gender differences among abused older African Americans and African American abusers in an elder abuse provider agency. J Black Stud 2002;32(5):557–73.
27. Cooper C, Selwood A, Livingston G. The prevalence of elder abuse and neglect: a systematic review. Age Ageing 2008;37(2):151–60.
28. Cooper C, Selwood A, Livingston G. Knowledge, detection, and reporting of abuse by health and social care professionals: a systematic review. Am J Geriatr Psychiatry 2009;17(10):826–38.
29. Burgess AW, Ramsey-Klawsnik H, Gregorian SB. Comparing routes of reporting in elder sexual abuse cases. J Elder Abuse Negl 2008;20(4):336–52.
30. Almogue A, Weiss A, Marcus EL, et al. Attitudes and knowledge of medical and nursing staff toward elder abuse. Arch Gerontol Geriatr 2010;51(1):86–91.
31. Tilden VP, Schmidt TA, Limandri BJ, et al. Factors that influence clinicians' assessment and management of family violence. Am J Publ Health 1994;84(4): 628–33.
32. Abbey L. Elder abuse and neglect: when home is not safe. Clin Geriatr Med 2009; 25(1):47–60.
33. Bergeron L, Gray B. Ethical dilemmas of reporting suspected elder abuse. Soc Work 2003;48(1):96–105.
34. Fulmer T. Screening for mistreatment of older adults. Am J Nurs 2008;108(12): 52–9 [quiz: 59–60].
35. Jones JS, Walker G, Krohmer JR. To report or not to report: emergency services response to elder abuse. Prehosp Disaster Med 1995;10(2):96–100.
36. Conrad KJ, Iris M, Ridings JW, et al. Self-report measure of financial exploitation of older adults. Gerontologist 2010;50(6):758–73.
37. Bomba PA. Use of a single page elder abuse assessment and management tool: a practical clinician's approach to identifying elder mistreatment. J Gerontol Soc Work 2006;46(3–4):103–22.
38. Conrad KJ, Iris M, Ridings JW, et al. Conceptual model and map of financial exploitation of older adults. J Elder Abuse Negl 2011;23(4):289–303.
39. Daly JM. Evidence-based practice guideline: elder abuse prevention. J Gerontol Nurs 2011;37(11):11–7.
40. Aziz SJ. Los Angeles County Fiduciary Abuse Specialist Team: a model for collaboration. J Elder Abuse Negl 2000;12(2):79–83.

Anxiety and Stigma in Dementia

A Threat to Aging in Place

Rebecca J. Riley, MSW, PhD[a], Sandy Burgener, PhD, RN[b],
Kathleen C. Buckwalter, PhD, RN[c],*

KEYWORDS

- Late-life anxiety • Stigma • Early-stage dementia • Older adults • Aging in place

KEY POINTS

- Behavioral and psychological symptoms (BPSDs), such as anxiety, appear in almost all persons with dementia (PwDs) sometime over the course of the illness.
- BPSDs are discomforting to the person with dementia; diminish his or her quality of life; and increase the risk for institutionalization, morbidity and mortality, more costly hospitalizations, and greater caregiver distress.
- Anxiety manifests through fearfulness, worries, restlessness, and irritability, as well as physical symptoms, such as racing heart and poor sleep.
- Anxiety is related to a number of adverse outcomes, such as depression, functional impairment, decreased self-concept, and insecurity, and can compromise the ability to age in place.
- Anxiety is related to stigma in persons with early-stage dementia.
- Stigma is a prominent concern among PwDs, resulting in shame, social isolation, and decreased quality of life.
- Assessment of stigma, anxiety, and associated depression is crucial in PwD.
- The Stigma Impact Scale, Rating of Anxiety in Dementia, and Cornell Scale for Depression in Dementia are tools recommended to measure these concepts, respectively.

Continued

Funding Sources: National Institute of Nursing Research, National Institutes of Health grant R03 NR010582-02 to Dr S. Burgener, PI.
R.J. Riley's dissertation research, University of Iowa, 2012 (3552027), was supported by a grant from the National Institute of Nursing Research, National Institutes of Health, grant R03 NR010582-02.
Conflict of Interest: None.
[a] Department of Gerontology, University of Nebraska at Omaha, 6001 Dodge Street, Omaha, NE 68182, USA; [b] University of Illinois College of Nursing, 210 South Goodwin Street, Urbana, IL 61801, USA; [c] Donald W. Reynolds Center of Geriatric Nursing Excellence, The University of Oklahoma Health Sciences Center, 2252 Cae Drive, Iowa City, IA 52246, USA
* Corresponding author.
E-mail address: kathleen-buckwalter@ouhsc.edu

Continued

- A number of interventions are available to treat anxiety in PwDs, including caregiver and health care professionals' educational programs, and pharmacotherapy and psychosocial interventions, such as modified cognitive behavioral therapy for PwDs.
- The stigma of dementia can be addressed by public and provider education, and in-home services.
- Older adults with dementia who transition between care settings and who live alone are particularly vulnerable to losing their ability to age in place.

Approximately 5.2 million Americans, or 10% of people older than 65, have dementia, with individuals older than 85 having the highest prevalence rate at 50%.[1,2] This number will likely continue to grow as the population ages,[3] and may be unsettling, as dementia is feared by many,[4,5] resulting in anxiety in persons with dementia (PwDs). This article focuses on anxiety, one of the least understood symptoms associated with dementia in community-dwelling older adults, the stigma of dementia, and the relationship between anxiety and stigma in dementia. When undetected and untreated, anxiety and associated stigma can adversely affect quality of life and the ability to age in place. The article begins by describing dementia-related anxiety. Next, based on research by the authors and others, the association between stigma and anxiety is examined. The article concludes with recommendations for assessment and treatment of anxiety and stigma in persons with dementia that will better allow them to age in place.

DEMENTIA-RELATED ANXIETY

Cognitive deficits have traditionally been the focus of treatment for persons diagnosed with dementia; however, PwD often exhibit behavioral and psychological symptoms (BPSD) that are disruptive to caregivers, and others in the environment.[6] Although they may fluctuate, behavioral symptoms appear in almost all PwDs sometime over the course of the dementia, regardless of etiology.[7] Anxiety and other BPSDs are important to consider, as they result in personal discomfort, diminished quality of life, premature institutionalization, increased morbidity and mortality, greater caregiver distress, increased emergency room visits and hospitalizations, and increased cost of care.[8]

Definition

There is a debate about the definition of anxiety related to dementia, as some symptoms of anxiety and dementia overlap.[9] Moreover, symptoms of anxiety, depression, and agitation also have similarities, causing further confusion about the definition of anxiety in PwDs.[9] However, a review of studies examining the difference between these constructs found more evidence supporting a distinct difference between anxiety and agitation.[9] Similarly, an earlier study examining behavioral syndromes in dementia (eg, hyperactivity, aggressive behavior, anxiety) found that these 3 syndromes were unique and should not be lumped under the construct of agitation.[10] Thus, the literature suggests that anxiety symptoms in dementia are identifiable, measurable, and treatable.[11]

Prevalence

Anxiety frequently occurs in PwDs in a variety of settings,[12] with caregivers reporting rates of 19.5% with clinically significant anxiety and 22.5% with subclinical anxiety.

About half of PwDs report occasional anxiety.[13] A pilot study found that 20% of PwDs who lived in dementia-specific assisted living and 100% of those who lived traditional assisted living reported 1 or more symptoms of anxiety.[14]

Symptoms and Related Outcomes

Anxiety is commonly exhibited through fearfulness, worries, irritability, paranoia, motor restlessness, suspiciousness, or day and night disturbances (**Box 1**).[15,16] Anxiety-related symptoms may also serve as an indicator of more challenging behaviors that could lead to unnecessary medication or harm to PwDs or others in the surrounding areas.[17] Other adverse outcomes associated with anxiety in dementia include greater functional impairment,[18] lower self-concept,[19] and attachment insecurity.[20] Type of dementia, disease severity, and gender also may be factors, as persons with Lewy body dementia demonstrate more anxiety symptoms than those with Alzheimer disease,[13] and anxiety occurs more frequently in men and persons with less-severe dementia.[15] Importantly, anxiety symptoms reduce the quality of life of PwDs, as well as their caregivers.[21,22] Further, anxiety can compromise the ability to age in place, in that physical or social environments in the community may become too much for the person with dementia to manage. Concerns regarding rejection from others due to the stigmatizing aspects of dementia can increase isolation as well. This may lead to avoidance of situations in which the environment is unfamiliar or where large groups of people will be present.[23] As a result, some activities that were once enjoyable to PwDs may become stressful.

Association with Other Behaviors

Anxiety also has been associated with behaviors such as wandering, sexual misconduct, hallucinations, verbal threats, and physical abuse,[24] with a higher likelihood of anxiety with each additional behavior exhibited. Similarly, excessive worry and anxiety in persons with mild, moderate, or severe Alzheimer disease was significantly associated with restlessness, irritability, muscle tension, and respiratory symptoms.[16]

Causes

Anxiety, as well as other BPSDs, may appear not only because of neurologic changes in the brain, but also as a result of the PwDs' inability to effectively express their

---

Box 1
Symptoms of anxiety

- Excessive worry or fear
- Refusing to do routine activities or being overly preoccupied with routine
- Avoiding social situations
- Overly concerned about safety
- Racing heart, shallow breathing, trembling, nausea, sweating
- Poor sleep
- Muscle tension, feeling weak and shaky
- Hoarding/collecting
- Depression
- Self-medication with alcohol or other central nervous system depressants

feelings, experiences, and personality.[23] For example, the ability to verbally communicate with others and comprehend what is being said in large groups may affect persons even in the early stages of dementia, leading to feelings of distress,[23] and expressive limitations may also lead to high levels of anxiety about everyday experiences, such as change or environmental factors.[22] Dementia-related anxiety also may be exacerbated by physical and emotional stimulation, physical illness, or situations in which the physical or social environment becomes overwhelming. Situations, including noisy chaotic environments, frustration with inability to identify objects, or inability to communicate needs effectively (eg, cannot identify or say the word of a wanted item), may lead to anxiety as the PwD's abilities to manage stress decrease.[25] Dementia-related anxiety also may influence outcomes on examinations and negatively impact performances.[26]

Sometimes specific triggers may lead to anxiety-related symptoms in PwDs, such as fatigue; changes in routine, caregiver, or environment; expectation to complete tasks beyond their abilities; overstimulation or understimulation in the environment; feelings of loss; illness; pain; discomfort; or being unsure of their surroundings and the expectations of others.[25,27] As a result of these triggers, PwDs may exhibit distressing behaviors to communicate their needs. It is important for caregivers (both formal and informal) to learn anxiety-related triggers to prevent escalation of undesired behaviors in times of stress.[28]

Insight and Anxiety

Persons in the early stages of dementia are those most likely to want to age in place, to have insight into their abilities, and to have higher rates of generalized anxiety disorder[29] and anxiety symptoms.[30,31] Specifically, they are better able to understand their diagnosis,[32] know there is no cure, and experience fears about how the disease will progress.[25,33] They also anticipate their cognitive decline and worry about future losses, dependency on others, and the reactions of others to their diagnosis.[34] Others fear losing their intellectual abilities,[34] and embarrassing themselves because of cognitive decline, such as forgetting who people are, or not being able to follow conversations.[29] All of these result in a perception of a lack of contribution to society.[34]

Feelings of insecurity and fear about the future may lead PwDs to become suspicious of the motives of others, fearing financial abuse or exploitation owing to their memory loss.[23] As a result of their awareness of cognitive losses and feelings of insecurity, some PwDs may overcompensate with hypervigilance and misinterpret environmental stimuli as dangerous.[27] Unfortunately, there is some truth to their suspicions, as PwDs are more vulnerable to exploitation than other populations.[23,35]

Relationship Between Stigma and Anxiety in Persons with Early-Stage Dementia

Stigma is a complex individual experience in which manifestation of diseases and social environments interact and in so doing affect personal identity and sense of self.[36] The degree to which a condition such as dementia is considered stigmatizing depends on a variety of factors: whether the person is thought to be responsible for the condition; the impact of the illness on others; and changes in ability and appearance associated with the condition.[37] Negative social meaning is linked to the person through a labeling process, and the person with dementia may internalize these meanings. Thus, stigma is potentially powerful because of the emotional responses created by the stigmatizing process.[38]

In 2006, the Alzheimer's Association launched an initiative that involved an advisory group of people with early-stage Alzheimer disease to bring first-hand experiential knowledge and serve as spokespersons, advocates, and advisors to the Association.

This group participated in a series of Voices of Alzheimer town hall meetings that provided the first nationwide forum for discussion about living with Alzheimer disease by people experiencing it. Those who attended the nationwide Voices of Alzheimer's town hall meetings reported the stigma of dementia as a prominent concern.[34] Some of these concerns resulted from the negative stereotypes and societal attitudes expressed toward PwDs[26] and reinforced in the media,[39] which can influence how individuals feel about themselves when diagnosed with dementia.[26] Others stem from behavioral symptoms that often elicit negative responses from others[40] and result in negative labeling of PwDs.[39] When people hear the word "dementia," they often have preconceived ideas and misconceptions of what the diagnosis represents.[34] As noted, individuals in the early stages of dementia are often aware of their deficits and, consequently, many experience symptoms of anxiety,[12,41] worrying about how others might respond to their diagnosis[34] or about embarrassing themselves.[29] Others experience shame surrounding their diagnosis and, therefore, may deny the diagnosis exists,[42] keep it a secret, or withdraw from social situations completely,[23] leading to social isolation, overdependence on family, and decreased quality of life. Thus, societal labels and attitudes impact how PwDs view themselves[43] and may influence their comfort with continuing to live in the community.

Similarly, the potential negative impact of stigma on PwDs was documented in a recent World Alzheimer Report.[44] The report noted that stigma can prevent affected individuals from acknowledging their symptoms and seeking the help they need to enjoy the highest quality of life possible, which typically includes aging in place.[44] Stigma can create situations in which even well-intentioned individuals and organizations become unhelpful; for example, by emphasizing the negative aspects of dementia and its symptoms and losses rather than supporting retained abilities in PwDs.

In a small study, people who had been diagnosed with Alzheimer disease in the early stages (n = 22) were asked to name their diagnosis. Most participants were unable to admit they had Alzheimer disease and identified several consequences that resulted from the diagnosis, including frustration and anger, self-blame, embarrassment, feeling cutoff from others, feeling useless, depression, feelings of loss, and feeling one would rather be dead.[42] These consequences may be indicative of the stigma of dementia and consequently influence a PwD's quality of life.[45]

Research Findings on Anxiety and Stigma in Dementia

As part of a larger, longitudinal, multisite (Illinois, Iowa, and North Carolina) study on Stigma in Persons with Dementia and their Caregivers, led by Dr Sandy Burgener, the investigators explored the relationship between perceived stigma and level of anxiety in 43 PwDs in the early stages of dementia.[46] Stigma was conceptualized as the stigmatizing responses of others, including labeling behavior (eg, not allowing PwDs to complete simple tasks once aware of their diagnosis), negative social interpretations (eg, beliefs that PwDs lack independence or societal contribution[39]), and suboptimal health care (eg, PwD is not taken seriously by his or her physician[34]). In addition, stigma included perceived stigma in PwDs that results from interactions with the external environment (eg, social rejection, internalized shame, isolation[47]). This study demonstrated a significant positive relationship between perceived stigma of dementia and anxiety levels ($r = 0.35$, $P = .022$); that is, as perceived stigma increased in persons with early-stage dementia, anxiety levels also increased. Social support, demographic variables, stage of disease, or mental ability did not mediate the relationship between perceived stigma and anxiety.

These results were congruent with the Voices of Alzheimer's town hall meetings discussed earlier,[34] where PwDs indicated the stigma of dementia had a negative impact on their quality of life. They also support other research showing that PwDs in the early stages tend to have awareness of the negative perceptions society holds about dementia[23] and may have internalized these negative societal attitudes, thus worrying about how others might respond to their diagnosis.[34] Findings from this study also support the need to develop and test interventions that have the potential to decrease perceived stigma and in turn reduce symptoms of anxiety in PwDs.

CASE STUDY—PART 1

Mrs Bernice Stasi is a 78-year-old widowed white woman who currently lives alone in a 2-bedroom apartment in a small Midwestern college town. Once very active in her church circle and bridge club, and an avid golfer, she seldom leaves her apartment these days, refusing all invitations from friends, family, and organizations she used to belong to because she "doesn't want people to know she is losing her mind." Approximately 3 years ago, she was diagnosed with probable mild cognitive impairment by her primary care practitioner, Dr Townsend. Her current Mini-Mental Status Examination score is 22. Bernice's only child, a son Tom, who teaches at the local college, lives nearby. He and his wife have assumed responsibility for most of Bernice's needs, including grocery shopping, housekeeping, and financial management of her affairs. Lately, he has threatened to put Bernice in the memory care unit of a local nursing facility, as she calls her son at work several times a day "just to be sure everyone is OK." The thought of being forced to live in a memory care unit with "those zombies" terrifies Bernice, and, if anything, escalates her insecurity and need to call people for reassurance. For some time after her diagnosis, Bernice refused to speak to or see Dr Townsend because she blamed him for giving her the diagnosis and "great shame" of dementia. But more recently she has begun calling the doctor's office several times per week to complain about her "fluttery" heart, trouble falling asleep, and feeling "shaky" when she walks around her apartment." Tom notes that his mother was "always a Nervous Nelly" but identifies recent increases in "nastiness," confusion, and losing things, all of which lead him to believe she needs to be institutionalized, "for her own good" and "our sanity."

Clinical Implications for Health Care Professionals

In general, nonpharmacologic interventions are preferred in the treatment of most late-life anxiety, as older adults experience changes in pharmacokinetics that may lead to medication toxicity, and many are taking an array of medications for other conditions that increase the risk of drug interactions. The first step in any treatment plan, however, is assessment. The following section recommends 3 instruments that nurses can use to assess depression (which frequently accompanies anxiety), anxiety, and stigma in PwDs. By establishing baseline levels, monitoring changes over time, and intervening early when any of these conditions become problematic, nurses can play an important role in helping community-dwelling older adults with dementia to age in place.

Assessment

For older adults, those with and without dementia, depression often accompanies anxiety, and both conditions can be debilitating, reducing overall health, quality of life, and ability to age in place. It is important for nurses to know the signs of anxiety and depression and to assess their older patients with dementia for both, making referrals to primary health providers and/or mental health professionals as indicated. One informant-rated instrument commonly used to assess for depression in dementia is the Cornell Scale for Depression in Dementia (CSDD), available from the cited reference.[48] The CSDD[48] is a validated severity tool that assesses for signs and symptoms of major depression in patients with and without dementia. Because some PwDs lack insight, have trouble articulating symptoms, or otherwise provide unreliable self-reports, the preferred method of administration is to first interview an informant (someone who knows and has frequent contact with the patient) and then to interview and observe the patient. Symptoms from the patient interview can often be filled out after direct observation of the patient, but should be supplemented by the patient's self-report. In the case of discrepancies in ratings between the informant and the patient interviews, it is recommended to reinterview both the informant and the patient in an effort to resolve the discrepancy. The final score, however, represents the rater's clinical impression on the presence or absence of each symptom, rather than the responses of the informant or the patient. Severity ratings of mild versus severe are made based on the symptom's: (1) degree of intensity or distress, (2) pervasiveness (ie, presence throughout the day), and (3) persistence (ie, number of days present in the past week). The CSDD is validated to rate depressive symptomology over the entire range of cognitive impairment.[48]

Each item is ranked for severity on a scale of 0 to 2 (0 = absent, 1 = mild or intermittent, 2 = severe). The item scores are added. Scores higher than 10 indicate a probable major depression. Scores less than 6 as a rule are associated with absence of significant depressive symptoms. A score of 11 or greater should prompt further evaluation of the patient for depression.

As noted, given the adverse outcomes associated with anxiety and stigma in PwDs, it is also essential that nurses are able to identify and monitor both conditions so as to intervene in a timely manner, help to prevent institutionalization, and maximize the PwD's ability to age in place. Two reliable, valid, and easy to administer instruments that nurses can use for this purpose are the Stigma Impact Scale (SIS) and the Rating Anxiety in Dementia (RAID).

Stigma Impact Scale

Perceived stigma can be measured using the SIS, developed and tested by Fife and Wright[49] and adapted for use with PwDs by Burgener and Berger.[50] The SIS is grounded in modified labeling theory[51] and is divided into 4 categories (social rejection, financial insecurity, internalized shame, social isolation). Social rejection measures feelings of being discriminated by others in society (eg, "I feel I have been treated with less respect than usual by others"). Financial insecurity focuses on financial problems individuals might experience as a result of their memory loss (eg, "I have experienced financial hardship that has affected how I feel about myself"). Internalized shame explores how much social rejection and financial issues impacted individuals' feelings about themselves and how they interacted with others (eg, "I feel I need to keep my impairment a secret"). Social isolation addresses feelings of loneliness, inequality, and uselessness (eg, "I feel less competent than I did before my memory loss"). The SIS yields a total score ranging from 0 to 96, with higher scores indicating higher perceived stigma.

Anxiety Level

The 18-item RAID scale can be used to measure anxiety levels of PwDs. The RAID is based on the total score of items 1 to 18.[52] The total score ranges from 0 to 54 and a score of 11 or more indicates significant clinical anxiety.[52] This scale was specifically designed to assess anxiety in PwD[52] by using caregiver or clinician-based observations of behaviors over a 2-week period. Items on the RAID can also be reliably and validly answered by PwDs in the early stages of dementia. The RAID is divided into 6 subgroups (eg, worry, apprehension and vigilance, motor tension, autonomic hyperactivity, phobias, and panic attacks[52]). Each question is rated as absent, mild or intermittent, moderate, and severe. The worry category measures the level of worry about various things (eg, worry about physical health), worry about cognitive performance (failing memory, getting lost when goes out, not able to follow conversation), and worry over insignificant matters. Apprehension and vigilance measures things such as sleep disturbances, autonomic arousal, irritability, and outbursts (eg, frightened and anxious; exaggerated startle response; short tempered). Motor tension (eg, trembling, headaches, body aches, restlessness, fatigability) is examined because the concepts of anxiety and motor tension seemed to be related.[53] Autonomic hyperactivity symptoms (eg, palpitations, dry mouth, shortness of breath, dizziness, sweating) are often reported by PwDs and are related to anxiety. Phobias are also reported in people older than 65, and this section of the tool addresses specific fears (eg, fears that were excessive, that did not make sense, and caused people to avoid crowds, small rooms, heights, and so forth). The section on panic attacks discusses the severity of symptoms of panic and asks PwDs to describe their symptoms (eg, feelings of anxiety or dread that were so strong that they thought they were going to die or have a heart attack).

In addition to assessing for anxiety, depression, and stigma, nurses also may wish to examine other stresses and changes in the life of a person with dementia that often accompany aging, such as poor mental and physical health and losses, that are associated with anxiety. For example, fear of falling, expenses associated with treatment for dementia and medications, being victimized, being dependent on others, being left alone, and death, can all increase anxiety in this population. Nurses should also consider alcohol or substance abuse issues, which may hide the symptoms of anxiety or make them worse. Investigating recent stressful events, such as the death of a loved one or pet is also warranted. Finally, nurses should inquire if PwDs have been treated before for anxiety and if so, ask about previous treatment, including medication and psychosocial therapies. If the PwD received medication to help manage anxiety, nurses should try to determine what drug(s) was used, dosage, side effects, and whether pharmacologic treatment was helpful. If the PwD attended therapy sessions for anxiety, the nurse should ask the person or an informed caregiver to describe the type of therapy, how many sessions, and whether it was helpful.

TREATMENT

Nurses and other health care professionals can play an important role in the treatment of anxiety and stigma, and are often involved in the evaluation of cognitive concerns. Therefore, it is important for them to be familiar with BPSDs[54] and to have an understanding of the progression of the disease.[55] This may help to guide treatment and to manage BPSDs (including anxiety), which often worsen as the disease progresses.[56] Treatment options can include medication, therapy, stress reduction, coping skills, and family/caregiver or other social support, some of which are briefly discussed in the following section. Nurses may directly intervene with PwDs and their caregivers or refer those they evaluate as being affected by anxiety and or stigma to mental health specialists, such as those in local community mental health centers or in the private sector.

A more general approach to management of anxiety is for nurses to help caregivers establish a routine and repetitive daily tasks, as this helps preserve cognitive functioning,[42,57] reduces agitation,[58] and provides PwDs with feelings of independence and self-esteem, therefore increasing their quality of life. Although the structure of daily tasks could become monotonous to family caregivers, it is likely that the management of distressing symptoms, such as anxiety, outweighs the boredom associated with this approach. Nurses can also provide support in a number of other ways as follows: helping the PwD acknowledge worries and address any fears that can be handled, such as talking about their responses to loss of abilities, or episodes of confusion/disorientation; encouraging them to express feelings and to talk with family members, friends, or spiritual counselors about such things as social isolation or fatigue; adopting stress management techniques, including meditation, prayer, and deep-breathing exercises; and avoiding things that may aggravate anxiety symptoms, such as large group situations, caffeinated beverages and chocolate, nicotine, over-the-counter cold medications and some herbal supplements, or reporting the anxiety-producing side effects of prescription medications. It is best to speak in a calm and reassuring tone of voice and to remain positive when talking to the person with dementia, and to encourage participation in activities, exercise, and pleasant events.

Educating Health Care Professionals

Interdisciplinary teams would also benefit from education about BPSDs, including anxiety, and possible ways to intervene when behavioral and psychological symptoms of dementia worsen. They should also be informed about potential triggers that escalate BPSDs; for example, that PwDs often become frustrated when they are unable to effectively communicate their needs,[22] so that symptoms may be decreased or prevented.[25,27] BPSDs are often points of stress with caregivers (both formal and informal) and may lead to premature institutionalization,[17] thus threatening the ability to age in place.

Caregiver Education and Support

Behavioral expressions, such as anxiety, can be stressful for caregivers and lead to premature institutionalization. Educational programs and dementia support groups can increase caregivers' knowledge of dementia, improve the ability of caregivers to cope, help them to feel less isolated in their experiences, and teach them to recognize behavioral symptoms. Programs that also identify mental health resources in the community for treatment of anxiety may allow PwDs to continue to live in their own homes and to better adapt to changing needs and conditions.

Anxiety Interventions for PwD

Pharmacologic interventions

Medication will not cure anxiety disorders but may keep anxiety symptoms sufficiently under control to allow the PwD to age in place. Although anxiety does respond to judicious use of medication, side effects are a key consideration in any geriatric prescribing, with all psychotropic medications in general, and benzodiazepines in particular. The types of medications primarily used to treat anxiety disorders are antidepressants, antianxiety drugs, and beta-blockers.

With antidepressants, symptoms usually start to resolve after 4 to 6 weeks, so it is important for the nurse to make sure the PwD is giving them adequate time to work. Antidepressants include selective serotonin reuptake inhibitors, such as citalopram, sertraline, paroxetine, and fluvoxamine, which have been found to improve anxiety, mood, and fear in this population, serotonin and norepinephrine reuptake inhibitors, tricyclics, and monoamine oxidase inhibitors.[59]

Anxiolytics, or antianxiety drugs, are sometimes prescribed when a short-term medication is needed. Benzodiazepines can be effective but should be prescribed only for short periods because of the risk of memory impairment, unsteadiness, and falls. Some older adults experience withdrawal symptoms if they stop taking them abruptly and there is a remote chance of addiction when taken regularly for a long time. Nurses may administer lorazepam (short acting, no active metabolites, available in tablet and liquid forms, average dose for older adults = 1-2 mg/day in divided doses to be adjusted as needed and tolerated) or oxazepam. Chronic anxiety is sometimes treated with trazadone or buspirone. Trazadone can be effective in treating sundowning behaviors (late day agitation/confusion) as well, if given in the late afternoon it is often the drug of choice. Beta-blockers, such as propranolol, also have been used with some success, as they can help relieve anxiety by preventing the physical symptoms that go along with certain anxiety disorders.[59]

Psychosocial interventions

Therapy or psychotherapy involves talking with a trained mental health professional in an effort to discover what may be causing the anxiety and how to better deal with its symptoms. Importantly, Medicare now reimburses for psychotherapy for PwDs.

Cognitive behavioral therapy

In cognitive-behavioral therapy (CBT), therapists help people change the thinking patterns that contribute to their fears and the ways they react to anxiety-provoking situations. A therapist can teach new coping and relaxation skills and help resolve problems that cause anxiety. Approaches include desensitizing the PwD to situations that trigger anxious feelings, and deep breathing and other relaxation techniques to relieve anxiety. Often modifications to standard CBT are needed to assist PwDs, as described in the following paragraphs.

The effectiveness of CBT as a treatment for anxiety in PwDs has been examined.[60–62] CBT skills, such as diaphragmatic breathing and coping statements, were implemented in 2 case studies conducted by Kraus and colleagues.[61] Skills were simplified so as to address comprehension, learning, memory, and application issues that may arise when working with PwD. To enhance learning and ensure understanding, PwDs were encouraged to repeat information learned back to the provider. Spaced retrieval was also used, whereby the PwDs were asked to correctly recall information over systematically increasing intervals over time (eg, recall after 10 seconds, 20 seconds, 40 seconds, 60 seconds, and so on).[63] Telephone contact between sessions encouraged skill usage and answered questions. Sessions were also shortened to 30 to 40 minutes because of fatigue in PwD. Caregivers were present during sessions and were encouraged to learn CBT skills, so they could remind PwDs to use the skills in their daily life. The 2 participants in this case study demonstrated reductions in anxiety after CBT was implemented, indicating that a modified approach to the skills might be helpful to PwDs in the early stages. However, because of the small sample and nonrigorous methodology, it is difficult to draw valid conclusions.

Peaceful Mind is a type of CBT designed specifically for anxiety in PwD.[62] There are 5 different modules discussed in Peaceful Mind, including self-awareness, breathing, calming thoughts, increasing activity, and sleep skills. Select behavioral rather than cognitive skills are emphasized, and only 1 skill is introduced at a time. Much of each session focuses on repetition and practice of skills, with visual cues and spaced retrieval techniques implemented to improve memory. After 6 months of treatment, most family members reported a decrease in anxiety on the Neuropsychiatric Inventory–Anxiety (86% at 3 months) with mixed results on other measures of anxiety.

CBT, implemented with appropriate modifications, seems to be helpful to persons who have early-stage dementia and who experience symptoms of anxiety. These studies provide hope that CBT might be a useful treatment for PwDs with anxiety. However, further randomized controlled trials with much larger samples are needed to determine effectiveness with this population.

Interventions for stigma

It is important for nurses and other health care professionals to be aware of perceived stigma and how this might influence PwD's willingness to seek treatment and talk about their challenges. It is crucial to understand that PwD, particularly in the early stages of the disease, are capable of making decisions about their lives and such things as where they want to live.[25,32] Indeed, PwDs are often open to learning new methods of coping, as these may ease disturbing symptoms such as anxiety.[64]

An overall theme that arose from the Voices of Alzheimer's town hall meetings were the issues of grief and loss. PwDs expressed concern that they would no longer be able to contribute to society,[34] and, that as the disease progresses, they might be forced to give up long-term careers. This in turn could lead to feelings of sadness, loss, and shame and a perception that they are no longer able to complete the tasks that were once second nature. Other participants in the town hall meetings noted that they lost relationships or were treated differently by their social circle.[34] Loss of relationships or status in the community may also have a negative effect on PwDs and lead to symptoms of depression or anxiety. Because some PwDs worry about burdening a spouse or family member with their concerns, individual counseling might provide helpful support in times of distress. As noted previously, nurses can make these referrals while at the same time encouraging PwDs to talk about feelings of sadness and loss and explore positive coping methods.

In the Voices of Alzheimer's town hall meetings[34] discussed earlier, persons who had early-stage dementia also discussed how the stigma of the disease affected their quality of life. They became socially isolated and felt disappointed with the lack of resources (eg, support and educational groups) available to them in the early stages of dementia. Thus, providing education and support services for this population is another area in which nurses can effectively contribute.

Public education about dementia

Nurses and other health care professionals may provide group, individual, or community-based programs that educate others about dementia and debunk stereotypes of PwDs as "the living dead" that can lead to their dehumanization.[65] It is important to provide accurate education to the public, as well as PwDs and their caregivers, about symptoms of dementia so as to address misperceptions about the disease.[66,67] Educational programs should also emphasize that PwDs in the early stages of the disease can often maintain a relatively normal life and continue to have joy and individuality.[66] Moreover, studies over the past decade support continuing insight and decisional capacity into the later disease stages as well. As a result of education about dementia, the public may begin to better understand the disease, respond more appropriately to PwD, and be more accepting of them in their neighborhood or apartment building.[4] Increased understanding of dementia may result in decreased stigma associated with the disease and improved quality of life among PwD.

PwDs have reported losing friends[66] because of a lack of understanding of the disease (eg, public is fearful they might "catch" dementia), and this negatively impacted their social and psychological well-being.[45] As a result, both PwDs[45] and those with mental illness[68] emphasized the importance of public education to reduce stigma.

Some expressed a desire to become involved in public education as a means of contributing and found this experience to be empowering.[34,68] The National Alzheimer's Association Early Stage Advisory Group[69] provided guidelines (**Box 2**) to PwDs to assist them in overcoming the stigma of dementia.

Individuals who feel stigmatized might benefit from joining together and forming groups that reject the stigma of mental illness and dementia.[70] This idea supports the expressed need of PwDs to connect with others who have been through similar situations[34] and would provide opportunities to learn more effective ways of coping.[70] The opportunity to be in a group that educates society about dementia or participates in research could instill feelings of worth and expand support systems, both of which are valuable to PwDs.[34]

Stereotypes about dementia are formed over a lifetime of negative experiences and contribute to perceived stigma.[26] After frequent exposure to these stereotypes, children form beliefs and values about what it means to have dementia. When they become older adults, they have internalized the stereotypes,[26] leading to feelings of shame and embarrassment about symptoms of dementia.[45] Thus, it would be beneficial for nurses and other health care professionals to develop educational programs about dementia for children that would help them to better understand the different stages of dementia, how to interact with individuals who have dementia (as many might have grandparents who have the disease), and hopefully decrease the stigma surrounding the disease. Resources such as "What's Happening to Grandpa?" by Maria Shriver are readily available and often helpful when working with children.[71]

Educating Health Care Professionals/Providers

As noted earlier, nurses often work as consultants to interdisciplinary teams (eg, physicians, other nurses, certified nursing assistants, social workers, physical therapists, occupational therapists, and others) in the health care field.[72] Interdisciplinary team members who work with PwDs would benefit from education about the stigma of dementia and how this might inhibit PwDs' willingness to share symptoms with others. As previously discussed, PwDs will sometimes deny their diagnosis and avoid medical care because they are uncertain about treatment options that could help them to age in place, and are unaware of medications[66] or other interventions that could help control troubling symptoms, such as anxiety. Specifically, the literature documents that the diagnosis of dementia creates feelings of anxiety about losing control and worries about how the disease will progress.[66] Sometimes, the fear of a dementia diagnosis is so strong that when PwDs (and their families) finally seek medical assistance, symptoms have become so serious that the person can no longer remain in the community.

Box 2
Guidelines for persons with dementia to combat stigma

1. Be open and direct

2. Communicate the facts

3. Seek support and stay connected

4. Don't be discouraged

5. Be part of the solution

Adapted from Alzheimer's Association. I have Alzheimer's Disease: Overcoming stigma. Available at: https://www.alz.org/i-have-alz/overcoming-stigma.asp.

Box 3 lists 10 general recommendations to help overcome the stigma of dementia as set forth by the National Alzheimer's Association Early Stage Advisory Group.[69] Although much more research on the effectiveness of specific interventions to ameliorate the stigma of dementia is required, the previously mentioned recommendations provide nurses and other health care professionals with suggestions for helpful strategies.

CASE STUDY: PART 2

Dr Townsend contacted the visiting nurse, Ms Carson, who had previously worked with Mrs Stasi and her family during her late husband's illness. He asked that they work together to address Bernice's anxiety behaviors that accompanied her early-stage dementia, and the debilitating stigma she was experiencing that contributed to her social isolation, feelings of shame and embarrassment, and that put her at risk for institutionalization. Together Dr Townsend and Ms Carson, in cooperation with Mrs Stasi, who "agreed to do anything not to be sent to that 'hell hole'" (memory care center), developed a plan that began with referral of Bernice to a psychologist, Dr Bertram, at the local community mental health center who specialized in the treatment of anxiety. The 10-week treatment sessions focused on helping Bernice to better recognize her anxiety symptoms and related behaviors.[73] Dr Bertram asked Bernice to complete a symptom and behavior log weekly and to bring the log to the next session. This enabled them both to monitor and discuss her levels of anxiety, activities or thoughts that prompted anxious feelings, and how she dealt with feeling anxious. By discussing the log and monitoring her feelings and behavior, Bernice began to develop some insight into how her calling negatively affected not only her own life, but also that of Tom and his family. Concurrently, Dr Bertram helped Bernice to acquire some basic skills to help manage her anxiety, such as deep breathing and problem-solving.[73]

Next, Ms Carson convened a family meeting to educate Tom, his wife, and Bernice about dementia, stigma, and the anxiety behaviors that commonly accompany the disorder. She referred Tom to a local early-stage dementia support group for caregivers and provided reading materials about dementia and its associated

---

Box 3
Recommendations to overcome stigma of dementia

1. Educate the public
2. Reduce isolation of the person with dementia
3. Give people with dementia a voice
4. Recognize the rights of persons with dementia and their caregivers
5. Involve persons with dementia in their local communities
6. Support and educate informal and formal caregivers
7. Improve the quality of care at home and in care homes
8. Improve dementia training of primary care providers
9. Call on governments to create national dementia plans (done in the United States)
10. Increase research into how to address stigma in persons with dementia.

From Batsch NL, Mittelman MS. World Alzheimer report: overcoming the stigma of dementia. Executive summary. Alzheimer's Disease International. 2012; with permission.

symptoms. Tom agreed to wait 6 months before revisiting the issue of moving his mother out of her apartment. Ms Carson made a contract with Bernice to attend congregate meals at the local senior center 2 to 3 times per week and while there to participate in an exercise class to help ease her tensions. She communicated these plans to Dr Townsend, who expressed his own frustration with Bernice's behaviors, but agreed to keep her on as a patient and see how her behaviors progressed. At the interim 12-week evaluation point, Bernice reported she "worried less," and did not feel "judged" by people at the senior center, many of whom she characterized as "worse off than me." The phone-calling behavior steadily decreased, as Bernice felt more confident and in control, and at the 6-month point, Tom and his wife agreed they would support Bernice's desire to stay in her apartment and age in place.

Interventions to Promote Aging in Place in Persons with Dementia Experiencing Anxiety

Strategies that foster early detection and treatment of behavioral and psychological symptoms associated with dementia are essential to enhancing aging in place. One such program, emphasizing care coordination and person-centered approaches is the Maximizing Independence at Home, out of Johns Hopkins University. In this program, a dementia care coordinator comes into the home to address a variety of care issues before the community-dwelling PwD spirals out of control and may need to be relocated. The coordinator maintains contact once a month or more often as needed, and assesses and refers for unmet needs and physical or mental health problems, such as anxiety. Importantly, there is access to an interdisciplinary team, including a psychiatric nurse and geropsychiatrist. The project demonstrated that people were able to age in place without sacrificing the quality of life.[74]

Finally, The Aging in Place project, sponsored by the University of Missouri–Columbia, has produced positive outcomes, decreased costs, and facilitated the development and evaluation of technology, although not limited to PwDs. The head of the project, Dr Marilyn Rantz, was named an American Academy of Nursing Edge Runner for the program, which relies on registered nurse care coordination, health promotion, and early illness recognition through Sinclair Home Care.[75] The goal of the project is to provide high-quality services at home, thus allowing people to age in place, and avoid or delay hospitalizations. Sinclair Home Care provides community-based care based on individual choice and autonomy. Services maximize each older adult's mental, physical, and psychosocial strengths. Costs of the program have never approached the average cost of nursing home care.[75]

SPECIAL CONSIDERATIONS FOR AGING IN PLACE: TRANSITIONAL CARE AND "LIVE ALONES"

PwDs tend to move back and forth between settings (eg, home, hospital, nursing home).[76] Transitions between levels of care are an important consideration for nurses in all these settings, as well as ensuring that PwDs have access to high-quality behavioral health services. This is especially critical for PwDs who may be temporarily residing in an institutional setting to ensure that they are able to return to their preferred home and neighborhood. As the process of transitioning across settings can, in itself, produce anxiety in PwDs, care should be taken to minimize the number and types of setting transitions. Another high-risk group is the more than 800,000 people in the United States with dementia who live alone.[77] About half these "live alones" have no identifiable caregiver, and are perhaps most vulnerable to being unable to continue to age in place safely and comfortably, regardless of age, income, or ability level.

SUMMARY

Both anxiety and dementia-related stigma are common among PwDs, especially in the early stages of the disease. Research by the authors and others has demonstrated a relationship between anxiety and stigma in this population. Nurses can play an important role in the assessment and treatment of these understudied and undertreated conditions in PwDs through psychosocial and pharmacologic interventions, educational programs, and support for health care professionals and caregivers of PwDs. These efforts can improve quality of life for PwDs and promote their desired ability to age in place.

REFERENCES

1. Alzheimer's Association. Alzheimer's disease facts and figures. 2013. Available at: http://www.alz.org/downloads/facts_figures_2013.pdf. Accessed October 25, 2013.
2. American Psychiatric Association. Diagnostic and statistical manual of mental disorders: DSM-IV-TR. Washington, DC: American Psychiatric Association; 2000.
3. Bloom BS, de Pouvourville N, Straus WL. Cost of illness of Alzheimer's disease: how useful are current estimates? Gerontologist 2003;43(2):158–64.
4. Corner L, Bond J. Being at risk of dementia: Fears and anxieties of older adults. J Aging Stud 2004;18(2):143–55.
5. Schwab M, Rader J, Doan J. Relieving the anxiety and fear in dementia. J Gerontol Nurs 1985;11(5):8–15.
6. Gitlin LN, Kales HC, Lyketsos CG. Nonpharmacologic management of behavioral symptoms in dementia. JAMA 2012;308(19):2020–9.
7. Cejejeira J, Lagarto L, Mukaetova-Ladinska EB. Behavioral and psychological symptoms of dementia. Front Neurol 2012;7(3):73. http://dx.doi.org/10.3389/fneuro.2012.00073.
8. Finkel S. Introduction to behavioural and psychological symptoms of dementia (BPSD). Int J Geriatr Psychiatry 2000;15:S2–4. http://dx.doi.org/10.1002/(SICI)1099-1166(200004)15, 1+<S2::AID-GPS159>3.3.CO;2-V.
9. Seignourel PJ, Kunik ME, Snow L, et al. Anxiety in dementia: a critical review. Clin Psychol Rev 2008;28(7):1071–82. http://dx.doi.org/10.1016/j.cpr.2008.02.008.
10. Hope T, Keene J, Fairburn C, et al. Behaviour changes in dementia 2: are there behavioural syndromes? Int J Geriatr Psychiatry 1997;12(11):1074–8. http://dx.doi.org/10.1002/(SICI)1099-1166(199711)12, 11<1074::AID-GPS696>3.0.CO;2-B.
11. Qazi A, Shankar K, Orrell M. Managing anxiety in people with dementia: a case series. J Affect Disord 2003;76(1–3):261–5. http://dx.doi.org/10.1016/S0165-0327(02)00074-5.
12. Ownby RL, Harwood DG, Barker WB, et al. Predictors of anxiety in persons with Alzheimer's disease. Depress Anxiety 2000;11(1):38–42.
13. Hynninen MJ, Breitve MH, Rongve A, et al. The frequency and correlates of anxiety in patients with first-time diagnosed mild dementia. Int Psychogeriatr 2012;24:1771–8.
14. Smith M, Buckwalter KC, Kang H, et al. Dementia care in assisted living: needs and challenges. Issues Ment Health Nurs 2008;29(8):817–38. http://dx.doi.org/10.1080/01612840802182839.

15. Calleo JS, Kunik ME, Reid D, et al. Characteristics of generalized anxiety disorder in patients with dementia. Am J Alzheimers Dis Other Demen 2011;26: 492–7.

16. Starkstein SE, Jorge R, Petracca G, et al. The construct of generalized anxiety disorder in Alzheimer disease. Am J Geriatr Psychiatry 2007;15(1):42–9. http://dx.doi.org/10.1097/01.JGP.0000229664.11306.b9.

17. Hall GR, Gerdner L, Szygart-Stauffacher M, et al. Principles of nonpharmacological management: caring for people with Alzheimer's disease using a conceptual model. Psychiatr Ann 1995;25(7):432–40.

18. Wadsworth LP, Lorius N, Donovan NJ, et al. Neuropsychiatric symptoms and global functional impairment along the Alzheimer's continuum. Dement Geriatr Cogn Disord 2012;34:96–111.

19. Clare L, Whitaker CJ, Nelis SM, et al. Self-concept in early stage dementia: profile, course, correlates, predictors and implications for quality of life. Int J Geriatr Psychiatry 2013;28(5):494–503. http://dx.doi.org/10.1002/gps.3852.

20. Nelis SM, Clare L, Whitaker CJ. Attachment representations in people with dementia and their carers: implications for well-being within the dyad. Aging Ment Health 2012;16:845–54.

21. Shin I, Carter M, Masterman D, et al. Neuropsychiatric symptoms and quality of life in Alzheimer disease. Am J Geriatr Psychiatry 2005;13(6):469–74. http://dx.doi.org/10.1176/appi.ajgp.13.6.469.

22. Smith M, Samus QM, Steele C, et al. Anxiety symptoms among assisted living residents: implications of the "no difference" finding for participants with and without dementia. Res Gerontol Nurs 2008;1(2):1–9.

23. Snyder L. The experiences and needs of people with early-stage dementia. In: Cox CB, editor. Dementia and social work practice: research and interventions. New York: Springer Publishing Co; 2007. p. 93–109.

24. Teri L, Ferretti LE, Gibbons LE, et al. Anxiety in Alzheimer's disease: prevalence and comorbidity. J Gerontol A Biol Sci Med Sci 1999;54A(7):M348–52.

25. Smith M, Buckwalter K. Behaviors associated with dementia: whether resisting care or exhibiting apathy, an older adult with dementia is attempting communication. Nurses and other caregivers must learn to 'hear' this language. Am J Nurs 2005; 105(7):40–52 Reprinted in: Clin J Oncol Nurs 10(2):183–91. Available at: http://search.ebscohost.com.proxy.lib.uiowa.edu/login.aspx?direct=true&AuthType=ip,cookie,uid,url&db=jlh&AN=2009129528&loginpage=Login.asp&site=ehost-live.

26. Scholl JM, Sabat SR. Stereotypes, stereotype threat and ageing: implications for the understanding and treatment of people with Alzheimer's disease. Ageing Soc 2008;28(1):103–30. http://dx.doi.org/10.1017/S0144686X07006241.

27. Boyd M, Garand L, Gerdner LA, et al. Delirium, dementias, and related disorders. In: Boyd M, editor. Psychiatric nursing: contemporary practice. 3rd edition. Philadelphia: Lippincott Williams & Wilkins; 2005. p. 671–708.

28. Hal GR, Buckwalter KC. Progressively lowered stress threshold: a conceptual model for care of adults with Alzheimer's disease. Arch Psychiatr Nurs 1987; 1(6):399–406.

29. Ballard C, Boyle A, Bowler C, et al. Anxiety disorders in dementia sufferers. Int J Geriatr Psychiatry 1996;11:987–90. http://dx.doi.org/10.1002/(SICI)1099-1166 (199611)11, 11<987::AID-GPS422>3.0.CO;2-V.

30. Eustace A, Coen R, Walsh C, et al. A longitudinal evaluation of behavioural and psychological symptoms of probable Alzheimer's disease. Int J Geriatr Psychiatry 2002;17(10):968–73. http://dx.doi.org/10.1002/gps.736.

31. Hargrove R, Stoeklin M, Haan M, et al. Clinical aspects of Alzheimer's disease in black and white patients. J Natl Med Assoc 1998;90(2):78–84.

32. Brechling BG, Schneider CA. Preserving autonomy in early stage dementia. J Gerontol Soc Work 1993;20(1–2):17–33. http://dx.doi.org/10.1300/J083V20 N01_03.

33. Sorensen L, Waldorff F, Waldemar G. Coping with mild Alzheimer's disease. Dementia: Intl J Soc Res Practice 2008;7(3):287–99. http://dx.doi.org/10.1177/1471301208093285.

34. Reed P, Bluethmann S. Voices of Alzheimer's disease: a summary report on the nationwide town hall meetings for people with early stage dementia. 2008. Available at: http://www.alz.org/national/documents/report_townhall.pdf. Accessed June 12, 2009.

35. Finkel S. Managing the behavioral and psychological signs and symptoms of dementia. Int Clin Psychopharmacol 1997;12:S25–8. http://dx.doi.org/10.1097/00004850-199709004-00005.

36. Goffman E. Stigma; notes on the management of spoiled identity. Englewood Cliffs (NJ): Prentice-Hall; 1963.

37. Reingold AL, Krishnan S. The study of potentially stigmatizing conditions: an epidemiologic perspective. Paper presented at the National Institutes of Health International Stigma Conference. Bethesda (MD), September 5–7, 2001.

38. Cumming J, Cumming E. On the stigma of mental illness. Community Ment Health J 1965;1(2):35–143.

39. Clare L. Developing awareness about awareness in early-stage dementia: the role of psychosocial factors. Dementia: Intl J Social Res Practice 2002;1(3):295–312.

40. Scheff TJ. Being mentally ill: a sociological theory. Chicago: Aldine Pub Co; 1966.

41. Mega MS, Cummings JL, Fiorello T, et al. The spectrum of behavioral changes in Alzheimer's disease. Neurology 1996;46(1):130–5.

42. Clare L, Goater T, Woods B. Illness representations in early-stage dementia: a preliminary investigation. Int J Geriatr Psychiatry 2006;21(8):761–7. http://dx.doi.org/10.1002/gps.1558.

43. Harris PB, Keady J. Wisdom, resilience and successful aging: changing public discourses on living with dementia. Dementia: Intl J Soc Res Practice 2008;7(1):5–8.

44. Batsch NL, Mittelman MS. World Alzheimer report: overcoming the stigma of dementia. Executive summary. London: Alzheimer's Disease International. 2012.

45. Katsuno T. Dementia from the inside: how people with early-stage dementia evaluate their quality of life. Age Ageing 2005;25(2):197–214. http://dx.doi.org/10.1017/S0144686X0400279X.

46. Burgener SC, Buckwalter KC. Examining perceived stigma in persons with dementia. Iowa (IA): US Department of Health & Human Services, National Institutes of Health; 2008.

47. Link BG, Cullen FT, Struening EL, et al. A modified labeling theory approach to mental disorders: an empirical assessment. Am Sociol Rev 1989;54(3):400–23. http://dx.doi.org/10.2307/2095613.

48. Alexopoulus GS, Abrams RC, Young RC, et al. Cornell scale for depression in dementia. Biol Psychiatry 1988;23(3):271–84.

49. Fife BL, Wright ER. The dimensionality of stigma: a comparison of its impact on the self of persons with HIV/AIDS and cancer. J Health Soc Behav 2000;41(1):50–67. http://dx.doi.org/10.2307/2676360.

50. Burgener SC, Berger B. Measuring perceived stigma in persons with progressive neurological disease: Alzheimer's dementia and Parkinson's disease. Dementia. Intl J Soc Res Practice 2008;7(1):31–53. http://dx.doi.org/10.1177/1471301207085366.

51. Link BG. Understanding labeling effects in the area of mental disorders: an assessment of the effects of expectations of rejection. Am Sociol Rev 1987; 52(1):96–112. http://dx.doi.org/10.2307/2095395.

52. Shankar KK, Walker M, Frost D, et al. The development of a valid and reliable scale for rating anxiety in dementia (RAID). Aging Ment Health 1999;3(1): 39–49. http://dx.doi.org/10.1080/13607869956424.

53. Yesavage JA, Taylor B. Anxiety and dementia. In: Salzman C, Lebowitz BD, editors. Anxiety in the elderly: treatment and research. New York: Springer Publishing Co; 1991. p. 79–85.

54. American Psychological Association. Guidelines for evaluation of dementia and age-related cognitive change. Am Psychol 2012;67(1):1–9. http://dx.doi.org/10.1037/a0024643.

55. Buckwalter KC. Alzheimer's/Dementia and behavioral management strategies. Iowa City (IA): University of Iowa College of Nursing: Webinar; 2009.

56. Kilik LA, Hopkins RW, Day D, et al. The progression of behavior in dementia: an in-office guide for clinicians. Am J Alzheimers Dis Other Demen 2008;23(3): 242–9. http://dx.doi.org/10.1177/1533317507313676.

57. Van Dijkhuizen M, Clare L, Pearce A. Striving for connection: appraisal and coping among women with early-stage Alzheimer's disease. Dementia: Intl J of Soc Res Practice 2006;5(1):73–94. http://dx.doi.org/10.1177/1471301206059756.

58. Alzheimer's Association. Alzheimer's and dementia caregiver center: creating a daily plan. 2012. Available at: http://www.alz.org/care/dementia-creating-a-plan.asp. Accessed September 24, 2012.

59. Expert Consensus Guideline Series. Treatment of dementia and agitation: a guide for families and caregivers. Postgraduate Medicine Special Report. 2005. p. 101–8.

60. Balasubramanyam V, Stanley MA, Kunik ME. Cognitive behavioral therapy for anxiety in dementia. In J. Moriaraty (Ed.) Dementia: Int J Soc Res Practice 2007;6:299–307. http://dx.doi.org/10.1177/1471301207080370.

61. Kraus CA, Seignourel P, Balasubramanyam V, et al. Cognitive behavioral treatment for anxiety in patients with dementia. J Psychiatr Pract 2008;14(3): 186–92.

62. Paukert A, Calleo J, Kraus-Schuman C, et al. Peaceful mind: an open trial of cognitive behavioral therapy for anxiety in persons with dementia. Int Psychogeriatr 2010;22(6):1012–21. http://dx.doi.org/10.1017/S1041610210000694.

63. Camp CJ, Cohen-Mansfield J, Capezuti EA. Use of nonpharmacologic interventions among nursing home residents with dementia. Mental Health Services in Nursing Homes. Psychiatr Serv 2002;53(11):1397–401.

64. Flood M, Buckwalter KC. Recommendations for mental health care of older adults: part 2: an overview of dementia, delirium, and substance abuse. J Gerontol Nurs 2009;35(2):35–47. http://dx.doi.org/10.1177/1471301207085364. Available at: http://search.ebscohost.com.proxy.lib.uiowa.edu/login.aspx?direct=true&AuthType=ip,cookie,uid,url&db=jlh&AN=2010179679&loginpage=Login.asp&site=ehost-live.

65. Behuniak S. The living dead? The construction of people with Alzheimer's disease as zombies. Ageing Soc 2011;31:70–92. http://dx.doi.org/10.1017/S0144686X10000693.

66. Devlin E, MacAskill S, Stead M. We're still the same people: developing a mass media campaign to raise awareness and challenge the stigma of dementia. Int J Nonprofit Volunt Sect Mark 2007;12(1):47–58.

67. Jolley DJ, Benbow SM. Stigma and Alzheimer's disease: causes, consequences and a constructive approach. Int J Clin Pract 2000;54(2):117–9.

68. Wahl OF. Mental health consumers' experience of stigma. Schizophr Bull 1999; 25(3):467–78.

69. Five tips to overcome Alzheimer's stigma. National Alzheimer's Association Early Stage Advisory Group. 2012. Available at: http://www.alz.org/i-have-alz/overcoming-stigma.asp#tips. Accessed March 10, 2014.

70. Link BG, Mirotznik J, Cullen FT. The effectiveness of stigma coping orientations: can negative consequences of mental illness labeling be avoided? J Health Soc Behav 1991;32(3):302–20. http://dx.doi.org/10.2307/2136810.

71. Shriver M. What's happening to grandpa? New York: Little, Brown & Company and Warner Books; 2004.

72. Cohen-Mansfield J, Jensen B, Resnick B, et al. Assessment and treatment of behavior problems in dementia in nursing home residents: a comparison of the approaches of physicians, psychologists, and nurse practitioners. Int J Geriatr Psychiatry 2012;27:135–46. http://dx.doi.org/10.1002/gps.2699.

73. Calleo J, Stanley M. Anxiety disorders in later life. Psychiatric Times 2008. Available at: http://www.psychiatrictimes.com/articles/anxiety-disorders-later-life. Accessed August 29, 2013.

74. Samus Q. International Alzheimer's Association Conference. Vancouver, BC, July 18, 2012.

75. American Academy of Nursing. Raise the voice edge runner factsheet. The aging in place project. Distributed at the annual conference of the American Academy of Nursing. October, 2012.

76. Callahan C, Arling G, Tu W, et al. Transitions in care for older adults with and without dementia. J Am Geriatr Soc 2012;60(5):813–20.

77. Alzheimer's Association. Alzheimer's disease facts and figures. 2012. Available at: https://www.alz.org/downloads/facts_figures_2012.pdf. Accessed October 25, 2013.

Nocturia in Older Adults

Implications for Nursing Practice and Aging in Place

Barbara W. Carlson, PhD, RN[a],*,
Mary H. Palmer, PhD, RN, C FAAN, AGSF[b]

KEYWORDS

- Nocturia • Sleep • Circadian rhythms • Symptom management

KEY POINTS

- Nocturia is an independent predictor of insomnia and deterioration of sleep quality and daytime function.
- Older adults with 2 or more voids a night have a higher risk of mortality.
- A targeted patient history, including a 3-day bladder and sleep diary, is important for identifying the cause of nocturia.
- In older adults with nocturia, interventions should focus on concurrent urinary and sleep symptoms.

INTRODUCTION

Nocturia is a common and bothersome symptom, which older adults seldom report to their health care professional.[1] According to the International Continence Society,[2] nocturia is defined as "the interruption of sleep one or more times at night to void, with each void being preceded and followed by sleep." Although associated with incontinence, nocturia is distinct from nocturnal enuresis, because bladder emptying does not occur during sleep. Particularly in older adults, difficulties in falling back to sleep has been associated with poor sleep quality, greater daytime sleepiness, increased disease burden, 1 or more falls, and symptoms related to primary sleep disorders.[3] Although there are several therapies for nocturia, it is becoming increasing clear that the effectiveness of intervention is highly reliant on understanding the linkages between disrupted sleep and circadian factors, which also influence renal and bladder function.

[a] College of Nursing, Donald W. Reynolds Center of Geriatric Nursing Excellence, The University of Oklahoma Health Sciences Center, PO Box 26901, 1100 North Stonewall Avenue, Oklahoma City, OK 73117, USA; [b] Division of Adult-Geriatric Health, School of Nursing, Institute on Aging, The University of North Carolina at Chapel Hill, CB# 7460, Carrington Hall, Chapel Hill, NC 27599, USA
* Corresponding author.
E-mail address: Barbara-Carlson@ouhsc.edu

Nurs Clin N Am 49 (2014) 233–250
http://dx.doi.org/10.1016/j.cnur.2014.02.009
0029-6465/14/$ – see front matter © 2014 Elsevier Inc. All rights reserved.

EPIDEMIOLOGY OF NOCTURIA

Although nocturia is the most common reason for nocturnal awakenings in all adults, the population affected by it increases with age. In a recent survey of US residents aged 18 years and older, nocturia affected 39.9% of adults between the ages of 18 and 44 years; the prevalence increases to 77.1% in those aged 65 years and older.[4] By age 80 years, the prevalence rises to 80% to 90%, with nearly 30% in this age group awakening 2 or more times to void.[4] Other studies show that in older adults reporting insomnia (N = 1424), nocturia is the primary cause of their disturbed sleep, occurring every night or almost every night,[5] and is the most common cause of deterioration in sleep quality.[6,7] Such findings highlight the need for greater awareness of the impact that bladder sensations and nocturia have on sleep, and via sleep loss, their potential link to a person's daytime function.

In addition to disrupting sleep, nocturia is associated with increased morbidity. Besides having twice as many doctor visits as those without nocturia,[5] people with 2 or more voids are more likely to rate their health as poor or moderate than those without nocturia.[5,8,9] In 1 study, poor health in women aged 40 to 64 years was positively correlated with the number of nocturnal voids, such that the prevalence of poor health approached 40% in women experiencing at least 3 nocturnal voids compared with 5% in those women who did not report any nighttime voids.[5] In addition, the need for toileting at night also places individuals at risk for falls,[10,11] particularly if they have disturbances in gait and balance, disorders of muscles and joints,[12] altered visual acuity, osteoporosis,[13,14] or altered mental state.[15–17] Insufficient lighting, extraneous furniture, and incomplete awakening when getting up at night are likely important contributors of nighttime falls.[17]

Other studies associate mortality with rising from bed 3 or more times per night to urinate.[18,19] Multivariate logistic models have shown an increased mortality risk among patients reporting at least 2 nighttime voids, even when controlling for comorbidities or correlates, including diabetes, hypertension, coronary disease, nephropathy, alcohol consumption, history of childbirth, and use of tranquilizers, hypnotics, and diuretics.[11] This relationship may in part be caused by an association between nocturia and other chronic conditions, such as cardiovascular disease, depression, and sleep apnea.[19–24]

PATHOPHYSIOLOGY OF NOCTURIA

Nocturia in older adults arises from a complex interaction between age-associated changes in bladder function and pathophysiologic processes that are commonly seen in older adults. As shown in **Table 1**, nocturia is attributed to at least 3 distinct pathophysiologic mechanisms: (1) diminished or nocturnal reduction in bladder capacity, which causes low volume voiding; (2) an overall increase in urine production (24-hour polyuria); (3) an increase in urine production only at night (nocturnal polyuria); and (4) sleep disorders, which aggravate the severity of symptoms.[25] Often, older adults are affected by 1 or more of these factors, and it is crucial that none is overlooked if a clinically meaningful reduction in nighttime voids is to occur (see **Table 1**).

Diminished or Nocturnal Reduction in Bladder Capacity

Diminished bladder capacity is a symptom of several medical conditions, including detrusor overactivity; neurogenic voiding dysfunctions; cancer of the bladder, prostrate, or urethra; bladder and renal calculi; and medications (ie, anticholinergics and β-blockers). In older adults, nocturnal reduction in bladder capacity is often the result of conditions that cause incomplete emptying of the bladder (primarily bladder outlet

Table 1
Differential diagnosis of nocturia

Condition	Diminished or reduced nocturnal bladder capacity	24-h polyuria	Nocturnal polyuria
Presentation	Urine production is within normal limits; increased frequency, small voided volumes (clear definition lacking), especially at night	24-h urine production exceeding 40 mL/kg body weight	Nocturnal urine volumes >33% of total 24-h volume
Possible cause	Overactive bladder Bladder outlet obstruction, including benign prostatic hypertrophy or obstruction Interstitial cystitis, urinary tract infection, bladder hypersensitivity, calculi, cancer, neurogenic detrusor overactivity	Poorly controlled diabetes mellitus (type 1 or type 2), diabetes Diabetes insipidus Hypercalcemia Polydipsia	Excessive evening fluid/ alcohol/caffeine intake Impaired circadian rhythm of arginine vasopressin secretion Renal insufficiency Heart failure Diuretic use Estrogen deficiency Sleep apnea Venous insufficiency, peripheral edema Hypoalbuminemia

Data from Weiss JP, Bosch JL, Drake M, et al. Nocturia Think Tank: focus on nocturnal polyuria: ICI-RS 2011. Neurourol Urodyn 2012;31(3):330–9.

obstruction), which could later lead to a permanent decrease in the storage capacity of the bladder (such as scarring from chronic cystitis, calculi, and detrusor hyperactivity). Thus, by the time older adults seek treatment of nocturia, they often show indications of both diminished bladder capacity and incomplete emptying.

The most common cause of bladder outlet obstruction in men is benign prostatic hypertrophy. With age, the prostate gland enlarges, leading to physical obstruction of the bladder neck. As the bladder neck becomes occluded, increased resistance leads to alterations in urinary flow[26] and, over time, causes urinary hesitancy, weak stream, extended micturition time (examples of voiding symptoms), urgency, and nocturia (storage symptoms).[27] Nocturia is the most prevalent symptom, with approximately 75% of men between 60 and 69 years old reporting having it.[27] Bladder outlet obstruction is less prevalent in women and is associated with anterior vaginal prolapse[28] and anti-incontinence surgery.[29] In general, prolapse is believed to be the result of pelvic relaxation as a result of multiparity, estrogen deficiency, or both.[30] In both men and women, bladder outlet obstruction can lead to overactivity as well as impaired contractility of the detrusor muscle. Combined with diminished bladder capacity, disruptions in detrusor muscle activity could lead to symptoms of overactive bladder (ie, urgency urinary incontinence and urgency). Incontinence associated with nocturia occurs when the nocturnal bladder capacity becomes overwhelmed by the amount of urine filling the bladder during the night.

Recent research has suggested that urgency (a compelling or strong urge to void that is difficult to ignore) is a major cause of both increased frequency of daytime and nighttime voiding and diminished voided volumes.[31] Thus, it is not unusual for individuals with nocturia to report symptoms of urgency, frequency, and other symptoms of overactive bladder.[32] Although the underlying mechanism for overactive bladder is not known, during urodynamic testing the patient often reports a strong desire (urge) to void during the initial stages of bladder filling, and uninhibited detrusor contractions occur.[31]

Twenty-Four-Hour Polyuria

The second category of nocturia is polyuria, defined as a 24-hour urine production exceeding 40 mL/kg body weight per day, with no day to night variation.[33] Often associated with conditions that lead to an osmotic diuresis, 24-hour polyuria is rare in older adults[34] but is a common symptom of poorly controlled diabetes mellitus (type 1 or type 2), diabetes insipidus, and hypercalcemia. In older adults, medications used to treat dementia, psychological or behavioral disorders, and pain are the most common cause of 24-hour polyuria (**Table 2**).

Nocturnal Polyuria

Unlike 24-hour polyuria, nocturnal polyuria is a syndrome that occurs most in older adults, whereby the usual day/night ratio of urine production is reversed.[33] In most adults, the volume of urine produced during the day is usually twice as much as that produced nightly. In patients with nocturnal polyuria, 24-hour urine output remains normal at 1000 to 15000 mL/d, but the day/night ratio is altered, with more than 33% of the total urine output for the 24-hour interval occurring at night. A bladder record that includes measurement of voided volumes is essential for the diagnosis of nocturnal polyuria. An example of a bladder record for evening and nighttime hours is shown in **Fig. 1**. The full 24-hour bladder record can be

Table 2	
Medications potentially associated with 24-hour polyuria	
Category	**Medications**
Polydipsia	Phenothiazines
	Anticholinergics
Central diabetes insipidus	Ethanol
	Phenytoin (eg, Dilantin)
	Low-dose morphine
	Glucocorticoids
	Fluphenazine (eg, Prolixin)
	Haloperidol (eg, Haldol)
	Atypical antipsychotics (eg, risperidone)
	Promethazine (eg, Sominex)
	Oxilorphan
	Butorphanol
	Lithium
	Demeclocycline (eg, Declomycin)
	Cisplatin (eg, Platin)
	Tetracycline
Nephrogenic diabetes insipidus	Amphotericin B (eg, Fungizone)
	Foscarnet (eg, Foscavir)
	Ifosfamide (eg, Ifex)
	Clozapine (eg, Clozaril)

From Weiss JP, Blaivas JG, Blanker MH, et al. The New England Research Institutes, Inc (NERI) Nocturia Advisory Conference 2012: focus on outcomes of therapy. BJU Int 2013;111(5):706; with permission.

Bladder Diary	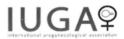

This simple chart allows you to record the fluid you drink and the urine you pass over 3 days (not necessarily consecutive) in the week prior to your clinic appointment. This can provide valuable information.

Please fill in approximately when and how much fluid you drink and the type of liquid.

Please fill in the time and amount (in mls, or ounces) of urine passed, and mark with a star if you have leaked or mark with a "P" if you have needed to change your pad.

Date/Time DD.MM.YY	Liquid Intake (ml)	Volume of Urine (ml)	Leaks	Pad Change

Fig. 1. An example of a bladder record. (*From* International Urogynecological Association. Available at: ww.iuga.org/resource/resmgr/brochures/eng_bladderdiary.pdf. Accessed March 8, 2014.)

downloaded at International Urogynecological Association (http://c.ymcdn.com/ sites/www.iuga.org/resource/resmgr/brochures/eng_bladderdiary.pdf).

The cause of nocturnal polyuria is not clear. Some studies,[35,36] but certainly not all,[37] have reported lower nocturnal antidiuretic hormone (ADH) levels. In others, the diurnal variation in glomerular filtration rate (GFR) is absent or even, reversed, with creatinine and sodium excretion rates higher at night than during the day.[38] The increases in creatinine and sodium excretion are often associated with higher nighttime blood pressure, which has led many researchers to suggest that both hypertension and nocturnal polyuria reflect a resetting of the blood pressure–naturesis curve that occurs with aging.[39] To better understand how to diagnosis and treat nocturnal polyuria, it is helpful to review what is known about the effects of aging and diseases on the diurnal variation in renal function.

Altered Diurnal Variation in Renal Function

In general, both GFR and renal plasma flow undergo diurnal variations, with GFR decreasing from 120 mL/min during wakefulness to as little as 36 mL/min during sleep.[40,41] In young adults, nocturnal urine volume, which includes the first void in the morning, is about 14% of their 24-hour volume; in persons older than 65 years, nocturnal urine volume averages 34%.[42] The diurnal variation in GFR and renal plasma flow is not neurally mediated, because it occurs in people who had renal transplants for fewer than 6 months and whose grafts are presumably denervated.[43] Although more research is needed, it seems that neither assuming a horizontal position[41] nor the fluid volume one ingests during the evening[44] influences the amount of urine produced in healthy adults at night.

ADH secretion is probably an important contributor for the normal decrease in urine production at night. ADH (also known as arginine vasopressin) is a peptide hormone released into the bloodstream from the posterior pituitary in response to stimulation of the osmoreceptors in the hypothalamus as well as arterial baroreceptors in the carotid sinus and aortic arch and volume receptors in the cardiac atria and great veins in the thorax.[45] An increase in osmolality, or a decrease in circulating blood volume, stimulates its release, whereby it acts along the length of the collecting duct epithelium in the kidney to reabsorb water via water channel proteins located within the epithelial cells (aquaporins) of the collecting ducts. In response to a large intake of water, osmolality decreases and ADH secretion is suppressed; less water is absorbed from the collecting ducts and the volume of urine increases.

In general, the ADH response to osmotic and baroreceptor stimuli remains intact with age. Compared with young adults, older adults also produce higher levels of ADH during the night than during the day,[35,36,46] but the nocturnal peak in ADH is lower[35,36,47,48] and the ability of the renal system to maximally concentrate urine[44] and to maximally dilute urine becomes diminished with age.[49] Other causes of nocturnal polyuria that most likely affect ADH or the ability of the kidney to concentrate urine include excessive evening fluid/alcohol/caffeine intake, inappropriate timing of diuretics, estrogen deficiency, and hypoalbuminemia.

Alterations in Sodium and Water Reabsorption

In addition to aging, nocturnal polyuria is a symptom of several conditions commonly seen in older adults, including persons with heart failure,[37,50,51] nephrotic syndrome,[40,52] chronic kidney disease,[53] and autonomic neuropathy.[54] All of these disorders influence fluid excretion by affecting sodium excretion, renal sympathetic activity, and release of atrial natriuretic peptide (ANP).

When blood volume is low, juxtaglomerular cells in the kidneys secrete renin directly into circulation.[45] Plasma renin then carries out the conversion to angiotensinogen by the liver to release angiotensin I. Angiotensin I is subsequently converted to angiotensin in the lungs by the enzyme angiotensin-converting enzyme. Angiotensin II is a potent vasoactive peptide that also stimulates the secretion of the aldosterone from the adrenal cortex, which causes the tubules of the kidneys to increase the reabsorption of sodium and water into the blood. Aldosterone also stimulates ADH secretion, which further increases water absorption at the collecting ducts and increases the volume of fluid in the body, which in effect decreases urine production and increases blood pressure. In healthy older adults aged between 60 and 74 years, baseline levels of renin synthesis and release are 30% to 50% lower than those seen in individuals aged between 19 and 29 years,[55,56] and they are considerably lower in persons with hypertension.[39]

In general, the diurnal trends in plasma renin follow closely those of serum cortisol and core body temperature, in that renin levels are lowest during sleep (between the hours of 2100 and 0900) and highest during the day.[57] The decline in renin begins just before sleep, and reaches its nadir between the hours of 2300 and 0100, after which levels begin to increase throughout the early morning hours.[58] In general, secretion of aldosterone lags about 2 hours behind that of renin.[59]

ANP is released from cells in the atria in response to stretching or an increase in blood volume, increasing sodium and water excretion by the kidneys at 2.5 and 3.5 times the normal rate, respectively.[45] Unlike aldosterone and ADH, the secretion of ANP does not seem to vary diurnally but, as discussed later, ANP tends to be increased in older adults with uncompensated heart failure. In heart failure and hypertension, as well as in persons with nephrotic syndrome, venous insufficiency, and autonomic neuropathy, nocturia occurs when sodium and water that accumulated in tissue during the daytime become mobilized at night or when there is use of diuretics and intake of caffeine or alcohol at night.

SLEEP DISORDERS AND NOCTURIA

The linkages between sleep disorders and nocturia is important, and several potential mechanisms link the 2 disorders. First, and most obvious, individuals with sleep disorders awaken more and often stay awake longer than those without problems. As a result, they are more likely to sense the need to void and then make a bathroom trip.[60] However, apart from such circumstances, nocturia is also commonly found in persons with obstructive sleep apnea,[61–63] and studies indicate that several interacting biochemical mechanisms may be involved. For example, sleep apnea is associated with decreased nocturnal plasma renin and aldosterone secretion, and treatment with nasal continuous positive airway pressure (CPAP) reverses these effects, as well as decreasing nocturnal diuresis and normalizing sodium output.[64] Nocturnal diuresis may be partially mediated through enhanced release of ANP and increased sympathetic tone,[64] although a role for ANP may be most readily apparent only in severe cases.[65] Although associated with heart failure, the release of ANP in sleep apnea may in part be caused by the high negative intrathoracic pressure during periods of airway obstruction and systemic hypoxia.[64–66] Unique to sleep apnea, increased urine production does not seem related to reductions in ADH, because CPAP has little effect on excretion of this peptide.[64]

LESS STUDIED CORRELATE OF NOCTURIA: DISRUPTED SLEEP AND CIRCADIAN RHYTHM DISORDERS

The timing and quality of sleep probably also play an important role in the severity of nocturia symptoms in older adults. Unlike younger adults, older adults tend to experience a shift in their sleep, in that they go to bed and rise earlier in the day.[67,68] In addition, older adults tend to have more frequent arousals and prolonged awakenings from sleep and have a higher prevalence of sleep disordered breathing and sleep apnea[69] and, once awakened from sleep, take almost twice as much time trying to fall back to sleep during the night than the young.[69] Older adults tend to spend more time napping during the day than do younger people,[70] which can affect both the time to fall asleep and once asleep, the maintenance of sleep. These disruptions in sleep continuity do not suddenly appear at age 60 years, but gradually start to occur during the middle years of life,[71] suggesting that sleep disruptions and impairment in sleep consolidation are not associated with aging, rather secondary to other ailments associated with aging.

Not surprisingly, in a national survey of adults aged 18 years and older, 75% of participants cited the need to go to the toilet as the most frequent reason for nocturnal awakenings,[72] with the proportion affected increasing from 39.9% in those aged 18 to 44 years to 77.1% in those 65 years and older. In this same report, the prevalence of other causes of wakening, like being bothered by a bed partner or child, thirst, dreaming, and spontaneous awakening, all decreased with age. Such observations beg the question as to whether older adults with nocturia awakened because of the need to void or whether they went to the toilet to void because they were already awake. Alternatively, it may be that altered sleep patterns affect the production of urine at night. In a pilot study with 3 groups of adults (those with overactive bladder, those with insomnia, and healthy controls),[73] the researchers found that in people with overactive bladder, nocturia was the direct cause of awakening, whereas adults with insomnia awakened for other reasons. People with insomnia had diminished bladder capacity (similar to those with overactive bladder), and the researchers suggested heightened sympathetic activation as a potential contributory factor.

Fig. 2 shows a conceptual model proposing the linkages between circadian factors, poor sleep, and upper and lower urinary tract factors that interact and contribute to nocturia. The shaded boxes indicate the factors, discussed earlier, that either increase the amount of urine produced (often associated with 24-hour polyuria and nocturnal polyuria) or decrease capacity to store urine during sleep. The open boxes and solid lines indicate the possible relationship between alterations in circadian mechanisms and symptoms of disrupted sleep and alterations in fluid excretion.

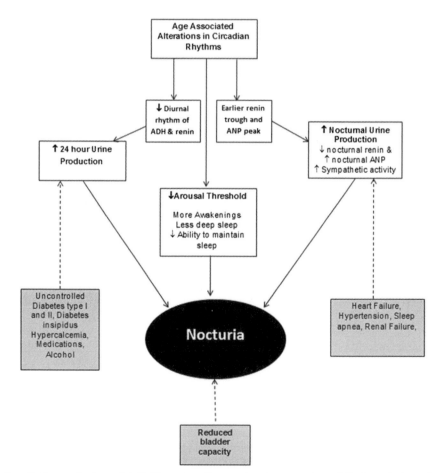

Fig. 2. Conceptual model linking circadian and urinary and contributory factors for nocturia.

The primary role of the human circadian placement in sleep-wake regulation is to ensure consolidated periods of sleep and wakefulness. In general, wake consolidation is achieved by a circadian signal that promotes wakefulness most strongly during the last part of the waking day. This arousing circadian signal opposes the wake-dependent increase in the homeostatic drive to sleep, which dissipates rapidly around the first 30 minutes of sleep. When the arousing circadian signal is advanced, sleep occurs earlier in the evening and individuals tend to get up earlier (often, between 4 and 5 AM). When this situation occurs, peak times for several physiologic arousing parameters (including core body temperature,[74] melatonin,[74,75] and cortisol[76]) are moved forward, from the early morning to the latter hours of the night. When this situation occurs, renin and ADH levels may be lower at night and lead to increased nocturnal urine production.

In addition, slow wave brain activity (a key indicator of homeostatic sleep drive) declines with age[77,78] and is often associated with an increased susceptibility to both internal and external arousal stimuli and a reduction in sleep consolidation, which allows the person to awaken at a lower level of stimulation. More fragmented sleep leads to increased daytime fatigue and less daytime activity, which together may contribute to less variability in GFR as well as levels of plasma renin and ADH.

CLINICAL ASSESSMENT

A comprehensive history and physical examination, including a 3-day bladder activity record and sleep quality assessment, are important for identifying the cause of nocturia (**Table 3**). Symptoms such as a weakened urinary stream and hesitancy, as well as a sense of incomplete voiding, suggest bladder outlet obstruction, especially in men.[29] A self-administered questionnaire, the International Prostate Symptom Score questionnaire,[29] has been validated in men and women.[79] It contains 7 items about urinary symptoms and 1 item about quality of life, and it can provide adults and their health care providers with information about the nature and severity of symptom. Women less frequently experience bladder outlet obstruction, sometimes occurring after anti-incontinence surgery; pressure flow studies may be needed to diagnose this condition.[29] Frequency, urgency, and bladder spasms are indicators of bladder irritation, and perhaps, infection. Gross hematuria might indicate a bladder tumor or stones.

Given that bladder outlet obstruction can be clinically subtle, one cannot rule out bladder disease in the absence of any of these symptoms. Urologic referrals may be necessary for more precise measures of urodynamic function, including tests of (1) urinary flow, (2) postvoid residual volumes, and (3) bladder pressure and muscle dynamics. In addition, transrectal ultrasonography can be ordered to determine prostate size in men, and for women, anorectal manometry and electromylograms of the pelvic floor and muscles, as well as measures of bulbocavernosus reflex latency, can be performed to assess pelvic floor weakness. A digital rectal examination can also be performed to detect fecal impaction, which can worsen nocturia symptoms.

Concurrent diseases, including obesity, diabetes mellitus, diabetes insipidus, heart failure, nephrotic syndrome, obstructive sleep apnea, chronic kidney disease, and autonomic dysfunction, should also be assessed. Orthostatic vital signs should be assessed to determine autonomic neuropathy. Dependent edema is often a sign of heart failure, but it is also present in other edema-forming states, including venous insufficiency and nephrotic syndrome. Abdominal assessment should consider the presence of a distended bladder or evidence of fecal impaction. Medications that might cause nocturnal diuresis, such as diuretics and calcium channel blockers, as well as intake of fluids, alcohol, and caffeine, should also be evaluated.

Table 3
History and physical

Component	Areas of Investigation
Urinary assessment	Lower urinary tract symptoms
	Voiding patterns
	Perceived bother
	Elimination of other urinary tract pathology
	Digital rectal examination to rule out constipation
	Completion of a 3-d bladder diary
Comorbidities	Obesity
	Heart failure
	Hypertension
	Diabetes mellitus/insipidus
	Renal disease
	Neurologic disease, including stroke
	Urologic/gynecologic disorders
Medications that may promote nocturnal voiding	Diuretics
	β-Blockers
	Calcium channel blockers
	Carbonic anhydrase inhibitors
	Xanthines (coffee, theophylline, albuterol)
	Antihistamines
	Cholinesterase inhibitor
	All drugs listed in **Table 2**
Sleep patterns	Usual bedtimes and wake times, number of times awakened from sleep, total hours spent in bed
	Daytime drowsiness/naps
	Reasons for awakening
	Usual place for nighttime sleeping, quality of mattress, room temperature, television, noise, lights
	Comfort in bed, pain, discomfort
	Pet or human bed-partners
	Ability to fall asleep after rising to void
	Anxiety, troublesome thoughts
	Snoring, restless sleep
	Wakening with shortness of breath or sweating
Fall risk assessment	Mobility, gait, balance
	Room lighting, pathways to bathroom, spectacles
	Falls history
	Toileting ability
Self-management strategies	What has been tried before and their perceived effectiveness
	Desired outcomes of treatment

The typical sleep pattern for each person should be explored not only to identify older adults with a sleep disorder but to determine the impact that nocturia has on their sleep. Information about usual bedtimes and wake times, as well as the timing of daytime and evening naps, assists in determining the shift in circadian rhythms and areas in which interventions for sleep promotion are appropriate. Because the risk of falling is an ever-present danger to older adults, conducting a falls risk screen, such as a history of previous falls, gait, balance, and mobility problems, is important. Recent studies have shown that the easily administered Timed Up and Go[80] test is a sensitive predictor of nighttime falls in older adults. Dim but adequate room lighting, cleared pathways to the bathroom, and easy access to eyeglasses also lessen a person's risk of falls.

Essential for managing health and aging in place, it is important to ask older adults about the self-management strategies that they use and the success of these strategies in reducing nocturnal voids. Obtaining a rating of how bothersome the symptoms are and the outcomes that the individual desires from treatment should also be explored. Validated tools are available, such as the International Consultation on Incontinence Modular Questionnaire for Nocturia–Quality of Life.[81,82] This questionnaire is a 2-item tool that measures the impact of nocturia on quality of life and outcome of treatment. The International Consultation on Incontinence Modular Questionnaire–Urinary Incontinence[83] probes the impact of symptoms of all types of incontinence on quality of life and outcome of treatment. Sleep disruptions can be assessed using the Sleep Functional Impact Scale,[84] an easy to administer, validated scale that addresses the impact of insomnia on patient functioning. When administered with a sleep diary, this instrument has the ability to provide a more comprehensive assessment of treatment response in clinical studies than a diary alone.[84]

TREATMENT OPTIONS

Initial treatment often involves lifestyle or behavioral interventions. Fluid restriction, including the restriction of caffeine and alcohol in the evening hours, can greatly improve symptoms.[85] Although not as effective in men with prostatic hypertrophy, reduction of fluid intake in the evenings is both an achievable and effective means of managing nocturia.[86] In some older adults, the benefits of fluid restriction should be weighed against the potential risk of other problems, including constipation and orthostatic hypotension. Information helpful to this decision can be obtained by having the older adult complete a 3-day bladder record, which includes information about frequency of bowel movements and blood pressure readings taken on awakening and before bedtime. Likewise, a change in the timing of diuretics, to late afternoon/early evening, may enable a full diuresis to be completed before bedtime.[87] Allowing excess interstitial fluid that accumulated during the day to mobilize through the use of compression stockings or resting with legs elevated during the evening may reduce nocturia associated with nocturnal polyuria.[87]

For some individuals, nocturia may have become a habit related to waking at night.[25,88] In this case, it is important to assist the person to maintain consistent bedtimes, and encourage activities that promote a calming bedtime environment to decrease waking during the night. In regions in which seasonal variation in sunlight exposure is greater or in institutions in which exposure to sunlight is minimal, melatonin, or even phototherapy, which restores the person's circadian time clock should be considered.[89] Melatonin may not only restore the circadian clock timing but could increase bladder capacity.[90] Of particular use in older adults are the newest types of prolonged-release melatonin receptor agonists.[91] Unlike other sedative hypnotic agents, these agents have an excellent safety profile, with a low risk of hangover effect or withdrawal symptoms.[92,93] Passive body heating[94,95] and warm foot baths[96,97] before bedtime, as well as gentle exercise in the early evening,[98,99] have been shown in some studies to shift circadian rhythms and sleep onset back in time.

Treatment of underlying medical conditions should also be addressed. Weight reduction should be encouraged, because evidence exists that obesity is associated with both sleep disorders and nocturia.[100] In women with urgency urinary incontinence and nocturia, pelvic floor muscle exercises and behavioral modification therapy could reduce the frequency of nighttime voiding.[101,102] Bladder retraining, timed voiding, and prompted voiding techniques can also be used for individuals with overactive bladder. Similarly, correcting hyperglycemia in persons with diabetes, optimizing fluid status in persons with heart failure, and reducing proteinuria in nephrotic syndrome can all lessen the severity of nocturia. Continuous airway pressure therapy in patients with sleep apnea not only improves hemodynamics and sympathetic output but also reduces the number of nighttime voids.[64–66]

Several pharmacologic agents can be used to treat nocturnal polyuria. Loop diuretics taken approximately 6 to 8 hours before bedtime induce a transient volume depletion, and once the diuretic effect diminishes, reduce urine production.[88] Other treatments, administering melatonin[90] or imipramine,[103] have been used with some success. In men with prostatic enlargement and bladder outlet obstruction, α-adrenergic blockers have modest effects in improving nocturia.[104] In women with detrusor overactivity and urgency urinary incontinence, bladder relaxant therapies such as oxybutynin, propantheline, and solifenacin have shown modest effect on symptoms.[102] However, the anticholinergic effects of these drugs often limits their administration in older adults with comorbidities. Caution must be used as all of these agents can precipitate acute urinary retention, especially in men with prostatic enlargement, and may be associated with acute cognitive changes in some older adults. In postmenopausal women, combination hormone replacement therapy reduces nocturnal voids after 6 months of treatment.[105] Topical estrogen creams improve atrophic vaginitis and can help to alleviate the associated symptoms of urgency and nocturnal frequency.[106]

There is some limited evidence that targeting sleep or insomnia may help to reduce nocturia for some patients; however, well-designed studies investigating this approach for treatment of nocturia are scarce. It is reasonable to assume that individuals with a true mismatch between the amount of urine produced overnight and the capacity of the bladder to hold urine overnight need to void, are good candidates for therapy targeting anomalies in urinary function. In the absence of such problems, targeting sleep itself may prove to be another viable treatment of nocturia in older adults.

WHICH CLINICAL END POINTS ARE IMPORTANT?

Although treatments are available for nocturia, the issue of which end points are most relevant has yet to be resolved.[107] In general, measures such as the reduction in number of voids per night, or percentage reduction in voids per night, are the most commonly used metrics for determining treatment effectiveness. Using this measure, studies indicate that those people with fewer than 2 voids/night experience minimal impact on their daytime functioning. It is reasonable therefore to argue that treatment that reduces nocturnal voiding to this level or lower is of clinical significance.

There are fewer standardized measures for determining the impact that treatments for nocturia have on sleep quality. The most common measure of the effect of nocturia treatments on sleep quality is the duration to the first void or first awakening from sleep.[101,102] Many of these studies vary in terms of how they define the start of the sleep period (ie, does it begin when the individual goes to bed, when they turn off the light, when sleep begins, or from the time of the patient's last void before they go to bed?), but once the individual is asleep, it is unclear if they include the time when the individual awakens for a reason other than the need to void, which might give a false impression of the fragmentation of the person's sleep. Perhaps reflecting the inherent problems with this measure, there is no conclusive evidence to determine how much of a change in this particular sleep parameter translates into a genuine improvement for the individual's health. Despite its limitations, the duration of the time interval to the initial void seems a reasonable and practical indication of the severity of sleep disruption in patients who have nocturia, especially if it is evaluated in combination with other measures, such as the number of awakenings for other reasons and the number of voiding episodes per night.

SUMMARY

Nocturia is a common complaint among older adults, and quality of life can be significantly improved if they do not have to withstand the bothersome effects of untreated nocturia. Although nocturia is often caused by some urologic disorder, sleep disruptions can and often do have a significant impact on the severity of urinary symptoms. Given the potential side effects of many of the pharmacologic agents used to treat both insomnia and nocturia, behavioral treatments should be explored first, keeping in mind what the affected individual defines as the desired outcomes of treatment. Working with older adults to set outcome priorities, monitoring symptoms, and adjusting treatment plans to minimize symptom severity are the keys to improving sleep and improving daytime function and quality of life in older adults.

REFERENCES

1. Chen FY, Dai YT, Liu CK, et al. Perception of nocturia and medical consulting behavior among community-dwelling women. Int Urogynecol J Pelvic Floor Dysfunct 2007;18(4):431–6.
2. van Kerrebroeck P, Abrams P, Chaikin D, et al. The standardisation of terminology in nocturia: report from the Standardisation Sub-committee of the International Continence Society. Neurourol Urodyn 2002;21(2):179–83.
3. Endeshaw Y. Correlates of self-reported nocturia among community-dwelling older adults. J Gerontol A Biol Sci Med Sci 2009;64(1):142–8.
4. Weiss JP, Blaivas JG. Nocturia. J Urol 2000;163(1):5–12.
5. Asplund R, Aberg H. Nocturnal micturition, sleep and well-being in women of ages 40-64 years. Maturitas 1996;24(1–2):73–81.
6. Bliwise DL, Foley DJ, Vitiello MV, et al. Nocturia and disturbed sleep in the elderly. Sleep Med 2009;10(5):540–8.
7. Cai T, Gardener N, Abraham L, et al. Impact of surgical treatment on nocturia in men with benign prostatic obstruction. BJU Int 2006;98(4):799–805.
8. van Dijk L, Kooij DG, Schellevis FG. Nocturia in the Dutch adult population. BJU Int 2002;90(7):644–8.
9. Tikkinen KA, Johnson TM 2nd, Tammela TL, et al. Nocturia frequency, bother, and quality of life: how often is too often? A population-based study in Finland. Eur Urol 2010;57(3):488–96.
10. Stewart RB, Moore MT, May FE, et al. Nocturia: a risk factor for falls in the elderly. J Am Geriatr Soc 1992;40(12):1217–20.
11. Nakagawa H, Niu K, Hozawa A, et al. Impact of nocturia on bone fracture and mortality in older individuals: a Japanese longitudinal cohort study. J Urol 2010; 184(4):1413–8.
12. Allain H, Bentue-Ferrer D, Polard E, et al. Postural instability and consequent falls and hip fractures associated with use of hypnotics in the elderly: a comparative review. Drugs Aging 2005;22(9):749–65.
13. Stone KL, Ensrud KE, Ancoli-Israel S. Sleep, insomnia and falls in elderly patients. Sleep Med 2008;9(Suppl 1):S18–22.
14. Stone KL, Ewing SK, Lui LY, et al. Self-reported sleep and nap habits and risk of falls and fractures in older women: the study of osteoporotic fractures. J Am Geriatr Soc 2006;54(8):1177–83.

15. Stalenhoef PA, Diederiks JP, Knottnerus JA, et al. A risk model for the prediction of recurrent falls in community-dwelling elderly: a prospective cohort study. J Clin Epidemiol 2002;55(11):1088–94.
16. Sterling DA, O'Connor JA, Bonadies J. Geriatric falls: injury severity is high and disproportionate to mechanism. J Trauma 2001;50(1):116–9.
17. Asplund R. Hip fractures, nocturia, and nocturnal polyuria in the elderly. Arch Gerontol Geriatr 2006;43(3):319–26.
18. van Doorn B, Kok ET, Blanker MH, et al. Mortality in older men with nocturia. A 15-year followup of the Krimpen study. J Urol 2012;187(5):1727–31.
19. Asplund R. Nocturia in relation to sleep, health, and medical treatment in the elderly. BJU Int 2005;96(Suppl 1):15–21.
20. Yoshimura K. Correlates for nocturia: a review of epidemiological studies. Int J Urol 2012;19(4):317–29.
21. Ferrie JE, Shipley MJ, Cappuccio FP, et al. A prospective study of change in sleep duration: associations with mortality in the Whitehall II cohort. Sleep 2007;30(12):1659–66.
22. Oztura I, Kaynak D, Kaynak HC. Nocturia in sleep-disordered breathing. Sleep Med 2006;7(4):362–7.
23. Parthasarathy S, Fitzgerald M, Goodwin JL, et al. Nocturia, sleep-disordered breathing, and cardiovascular morbidity in a community-based cohort. PLoS One 2012;7(2):e30969.
24. Lightner DJ, Krambeck AE, Jacobson DJ, et al. Nocturia is associated with an increased risk of coronary heart disease and death. BJU Int 2012;110(6):848–53.
25. Ancoli-Israel S, Bliwise DL, Norgaard JP. The effect of nocturia on sleep. Sleep Med Rev 2011;15(2):91–7.
26. McVary KT, Roehrborn CG, Avins AL, et al. Update on AUA guideline on the management of benign prostatic hyperplasia. J Urol 2011;185(5):1793–803.
27. Wei JT, Calhoun E, Jacobsen SJ. Urologic diseases in America project: benign prostatic hyperplasia. J Urol 2008;179(5 Suppl):S75–80.
28. Dancz CE, Ozel B. Is there a pelvic organ prolapse threshold that predicts bladder outflow obstruction? Int Urogynecol J 2011;22(7):863–8.
29. Lemack GE. Urodynamic assessment of bladder-outlet obstruction in women. Nat Clin Pract Urol 2006;3(1):38–44.
30. Haylen BT, de Ridder D, Freeman RM, et al. An International Urogynecological Association (IUGA)/International Continence Society (ICS) joint report on the terminology for female pelvic floor dysfunction. Neurourol Urodyn 2010;29(1):4–20.
31. Abrams P, Chapple CR, Junemann KP, et al. Urinary urgency: a review of its assessment as the key symptom of the overactive bladder syndrome. World J Urol 2012;30(3):385–92.
32. Abrams P, Cardozo L, Fall M, et al. The standardisation of terminology of lower urinary tract function: report from the Standardisation Sub-committee of the International Continence Society. Neurourol Urodyn 2002;21(2):167–78.
33. Weiss JP, Bosch JL, Drake M, et al. Nocturia Think Tank: focus on nocturnal polyuria: ICI-RS 2011. Neurourol Urodyn 2012;31(3):330–9.
34. Asplund R. Pharmacotherapy for nocturia in the elderly patient. Drugs Aging 2007;24(4):325–43.
35. Asplund R, Aberg H. Diurnal variation in the levels of antidiuretic hormone in the elderly. J Intern Med 1991;229(2):131–4.
36. Bodo G, Gontero P, Casetta G, et al. Circadian antidiuretic hormone variation in elderly men complaining of persistent nocturia after urinary flow obstruction removal. Scand J Urol Nephrol 1998;32(5):320–4.

37. Hirayama A, Torimoto K, Yamada A, et al. Relationship between nocturnal urine volume, leg edema, and urinary antidiuretic hormone in older men. Urology 2011;77(6):1426–31.
38. Fujii T, Uzu T, Nishimura M, et al. Circadian rhythm of natriuresis is disturbed in nondipper type of essential hypertension. Am J Kidney Dis 1999;33(1):29–35.
39. Feldstein CA. Nocturia in arterial hypertension: a prevalent, underreported, and sometimes underestimated association. J Am Soc Hypertens 2013;7(1):75–84.
40. Voogel AJ, Koopman MG, Hart AA, et al. Circadian rhythms in systemic hemodynamics and renal function in healthy subjects and patients with nephrotic syndrome. Kidney Int 2001;59(5):1873–80.
41. Koopman MG, Koomen GC, Krediet RT, et al. Circadian rhythm of glomerular filtration rate in normal individuals. Clin Sci 1989;77(1):105–11.
42. Kirkland JL, Lye M, Levy DW, et al. Patterns of urine flow and electrolyte excretion in healthy elderly people. BMJ 1983;287(6406):1665–7.
43. Buijsen JG, van Acker BA, Koomen GC, et al. Circadian rhythm of glomerular filtration rate in patients after kidney transplantation. Nephrol Dial Transplant 1994;9(9):1330–3.
44. Rowe JW, Shock NW, DeFronzo RA. The influence of age on the renal response to water deprivation in man. Nephron 1976;17(4):270–8.
45. Jequier E, Constant F. Water as an essential nutrient: the physiological basis of hydration. Eur J Clin Nutr 2010;64(2):115–23.
46. George CP, Messerli FH, Genest J, et al. Diurnal variation of plasma vasopressin in man. J Clin Endocrinol Metab 1975;41(2):332–8.
47. Moon DG, Jin MH, Lee JG, et al. Antidiuretic hormone in elderly male patients with severe nocturia: a circadian study. BJU Int 2004;94(4):571–5.
48. Davis PJ, Davis FB. Water excretion in the elderly. Endocrinol Metab Clin North Am 1987;16(4):867–75.
49. Madersbacher S, Pycha A, Schatzl G, et al. The aging lower urinary tract: a comparative urodynamic study of men and women. Urology 1998;51(2):206–12.
50. Hayes D Jr, Anstead MI, Ho J, et al. Insomnia and chronic heart failure. Heart Fail Rev 2009;14(3):171–82.
51. Redeker NS, Adams L, Berkowitz R, et al. Nocturia, sleep and daytime function in stable heart failure. J Card Fail 2012;18(7):569–75.
52. Koopman MG, Krediet RT, Zuyderhoudt FJ, et al. A circadian rhythm of proteinuria in patients with a nephrotic syndrome. Clin Sci 1985;69(4):395–401.
53. Hillier P, Knapp MS, Cove-Smith R. Circadian variations in urine excretion in chronic renal failure. Q J Med 1980;49(196):461–78.
54. Wilcox CS, Aminoff MJ, Penn W. Basis of nocturnal polyuria in patients with autonomic failure. J Neurol Neurosurg Psychiatr 1974;37(6):677–84.
55. Weidmann P, De Myttenaere-Bursztein S, Maxwell MH, et al. Effect on aging on plasma renin and aldosterone in normal man. Kidney Int 1975;8(5):325–33.
56. Weidmann P, de Chatel R, Schiffmann A, et al. Interrelations between age and plasma renin, aldosterone and cortisol, urinary catecholamines, and the body sodium/volume state in normal man. Klin Wochenschr 1977;55(15):725–33.
57. Portaluppi F, Bagni B, degli Uberti E, et al. Circadian rhythms of atrial natriuretic peptide, renin, aldosterone, cortisol, blood pressure and heart rate in normal and hypertensive subjects. J Hypertens 1990;8(1):85–95.
58. Stern N, Sowers JR, McGinty D, et al. Circadian rhythm of plasma renin activity in older normal and essential hypertensive men: relation with inactive renin, aldosterone, cortisol and REM sleep. J Hypertens 1986;4(5):543–50.

59. Hurwitz S, Cohen RJ, Williams GH. Diurnal variation of aldosterone and plasma renin activity: timing relation to melatonin and cortisol and consistency after prolonged bed rest. J Appl Phys 2004;96(4):1406–14.
60. Helfand BT, McVary KT, Meleth S, et al. The relationship between lower urinary tract symptom severity and sleep disturbance in the CAMUS trial. J Urol 2011; 185(6):2223–8.
61. Gjorup PH, Sadauskiene L, Wessels J, et al. Increased nocturnal sodium excretion in obstructive sleep apnoea. Relation to nocturnal change in diastolic blood pressure. Scand J Clin Lab Invest 2008;68(1):11–21.
62. Ljunggren M, Lindahl B, Theorell-Haglow J, et al. Association between obstructive sleep apnea and elevated levels of type B natriuretic peptide in a community-based sample of women. Sleep 2012;35(11):1521–7.
63. Kita H, Ohi M, Chin K, et al. The nocturnal secretion of cardiac natriuretic peptides during obstructive sleep apnoea and its response to therapy with nasal continuous positive airway pressure. J Sleep Res 1998;7(3):199–207.
64. Rodenstein DO, D'Odemont JP, Pieters T, et al. Diurnal and nocturnal diuresis and natriuresis in obstructive sleep apnea. Effects of nasal continuous positive airway pressure therapy. Am Rev Respir Dis 1992;145(6):1367–71.
65. Krieger J, Follenius M, Sforza E, et al. Effects of treatment with nasal continuous positive airway pressure on atrial natriuretic peptide and arginine vasopressin release during sleep in patients with obstructive sleep apnoea. Clin Sci 1991; 80(5):443–9.
66. Krieger J, Laks L, Wilcox I, et al. Atrial natriuretic peptide release during sleep in patients with obstructive sleep apnoea before and during treatment with nasal continuous positive airway pressure. Clin Sci 1989;77(4):407–11.
67. Pace-Schott EF, Spencer RM. Age-related changes in the cognitive function of sleep. Prog Brain Res 2011;191:75–89.
68. Cajochen C, Munch M, Knoblauch V, et al. Age-related changes in the circadian and homeostatic regulation of human sleep. Chronobiol Int 2006;23(1–2):461–74.
69. Bliwise DL. Sleep in normal aging and dementia. Sleep 1993;16(1):40–81.
70. Goldman SE, Hall M, Boudreau R, et al. Association between nighttime sleep and napping in older adults. Sleep 2008;31(5):733–40.
71. Carrier J, Land S, Buysse DJ, et al. The effects of age and gender on sleep EEG power spectral density in the middle years of life (ages 20-60 years old). Psychophysiology 2001;38(2):232–42.
72. Ohayon MM. Nocturnal awakenings and comorbid disorders in the American general population. J Psychiatr Res 2008;43(1):48–54.
73. Preud'homme XA, Amundsen CL, Webster GD, et al. Comparison of diary-derived bladder and sleep measurements across OAB individuals, primary insomniacs, and healthy controls. Int Urogynecol J 2013;24(3):501–8.
74. Dijk DJ, Duffy JF, Riel E, et al. Ageing and the circadian and homeostatic regulation of human sleep during forced desynchrony of rest, melatonin and temperature rhythms. J Physiol 1999;516(Pt 2):611–27.
75. Duffy JF, Dijk DJ, Hall EF, et al. Relationship of endogenous circadian melatonin and temperature rhythms to self-reported preference for morning or evening activity in young and older people. J Investig Med 1999;47(3):141–50.
76. Ferrari E, Casarotti D, Muzzoni B, et al. Age-related changes of the adrenal secretory pattern: possible role in pathological brain aging. Brain Res Rev 2001;37(1–3):294–300.
77. Dijk DJ, Groeger JA, Stanley N, et al. Age-related reduction in daytime sleep propensity and nocturnal slow wave sleep. Sleep 2010;33(2):211–23.

78. Viola AU, Chellappa SL, Archer SN, et al. Interindividual differences in circadian rhythmicity and sleep homeostasis in older people: effect of a PER3 polymorphism. Neurobiol Aging 2012;33(5):1010.e17–27.
79. Barry MJ, Fowler FJ Jr, O'Leary MP, et al. The American Urological Association symptom index for benign prostatic hyperplasia. The Measurement Committee of the American Urological Association. J Urol 1992;148(5):1549–57.
80. Lee J, Geller AI, Strasser DC. Analytical review: focus on fall screening assessments. PM R 2013;5(7):609–21.
81. Simaioforidis V, Papatsoris AG, Chrisofos M, et al. Tamsulosin versus transurethral resection of the prostate: effect on nocturia as a result of benign prostatic hyperplasia. Int J Urol 2011;18(3):243–8.
82. Donovan JL, Abrams P, Peters TJ, et al. The ICS-'BPH' Study: the psychometric validity and reliability of the ICSmale questionnaire. Br J Urol 1996;77(4):554–62.
83. Avery K, Donovan J, Peters TJ, et al. ICIQ: a brief and robust measure for evaluating the symptoms and impact of urinary incontinence. Neurourol Urodyn 2004;23(4):322–30.
84. Bell C, McLeod LD, Nelson LM, et al. Development and psychometric evaluation of a new patient-reported outcome instrument measuring the functional impact of insomnia. Qual Life Res 2011;20(9):1457–68.
85. Van Kerrebroeck P, Abrams P, Chaikin D, et al. The standardization of terminology in nocturia: report from the standardization subcommittee of the International Continence Society. BJU Int 2002;90(Suppl 3):11–5.
86. Hashim H, Abrams P. How should patients with an overactive bladder manipulate their fluid intake? BJU Int 2008;102(1):62–6.
87. Marinkovic SP, Gillen LM, Stanton SL. Managing nocturia. BMJ 2004;328(7447):1063–6.
88. Reynard JM, Cannon A, Abrams P. Conservative management of nocturia in adults (protocol). Cochrane Database Syst Rev 2004;(1):CD004669.
89. Sugaya K, Nishijima S, Miyazato M, et al. Effects of melatonin and rilmazafone on nocturia in the elderly. J Int Med Res 2007;35(5):685–91.
90. Drake MJ, Mills IW, Noble JG. Melatonin pharmacotherapy for nocturia in men with benign prostatic enlargement. J Urol 2004;171(3):1199–202.
91. Lemoine P, Garfinkel D, Laudon M, et al. Prolonged-release melatonin for insomnia–an open-label long-term study of efficacy, safety, and withdrawal. Ther Clin Risk Manag 2011;7:301–11.
92. Wade AG, Crawford G, Ford I, et al. Prolonged release melatonin in the treatment of primary insomnia: evaluation of the age cut-off for short- and long-term response. Curr Med Res Opin 2011;27(1):87–98.
93. Roth T, Seiden D, Wang-Weigand S, et al. A 2-night, 3-period, crossover study of ramelteon's efficacy and safety in older adults with chronic insomnia. Curr Med Res Opin 2007;23(5):1005–14.
94. Liao WC. Effects of passive body heating on body temperature and sleep regulation in the elderly: a systematic review. Int J Nurs Stud 2002;39(8):803–10.
95. Dorsey CM, Lukas SE, Teicher MH, et al. Effects of passive body heating on the sleep of older female insomniacs. J Geriatr Psychiatry Neurol 1996;9(2):83–90.
96. Liao WC, Chiu MJ, Landis CA. A warm footbath before bedtime and sleep in older Taiwanese with sleep disturbance. Res Nurs Health 2008;31(5):514–28.
97. Liao WC, Landis CA, Lentz MJ, et al. Effect of foot bathing on distal-proximal skin temperature gradient in elders. Int J Nurs Stud 2005;42(7):717–22.

98. Van Reeth O, Sturis J, Byrne MM, et al. Nocturnal exercise phase delays circa-dian rhythms of melatonin and thyrotropin secretion in normal men. Am J Phys 1994;266(6 Pt 1):E964–74.

99. Bukowski EL, Conway A, Glentz LA, et al. The effect of iyengar yoga and strengthening exercises for people living with osteoarthritis of the knee: a case series. Int Q Community Health Educ 2006;26(3):287–305.

100. Cornu JN, Abrams P, Chapple CR, et al. A contemporary assessment of noctu-ria: definition, epidemiology, pathophysiology, and management–a systematic review and meta-analysis. Eur Urol 2012;62(5):877–90.

101. Fantl JA. Behavioral intervention for community-dwelling individuals with urinary incontinence. Urol 1998;51(2A Suppl):30–4.

102. Johnson TM 2nd, Burgio KL, Redden DT, et al. Effects of behavioral and drug therapy on nocturia in older incontinent women. J Am Geriatr Soc 2005;53(5): 846–50.

103. Hunsballe JM, Rittig S, Pedersen EB, et al. Single dose imipramine reduces nocturnal urine output in patients with nocturnal enuresis and nocturnal polyuria. J Urol 1997;158(3 Pt 1):830–6.

104. Johnson TM 2nd, Jones K, Williford WO, et al. Changes in nocturia from medical treatment of benign prostatic hyperplasia: secondary analysis of the Depart-ment of Veterans Affairs Cooperative Study Trial. J Urol 2003;170(1):145–8.

105. Long CY, Liu CM, Hsu SC, et al. A randomized comparative study of the effects of oral and topical estrogen therapy on the lower urinary tract of hysterecto-mized postmenopausal women. Fertil Steril 2006;85(1):155–60.

106. Cardozo L, Robinson D. Special considerations in premenopausal and post-menopausal women with symptoms of overactive bladder. Urology 2002;60(5 Suppl 1):64–71.

107. Weiss JP, Blaivas JG, Blanker MH, et al. The New England Research Institutes, Inc. (NERI) Nocturia Advisory Conference 2012: focus on outcomes of therapy. BJU Int 2013;111(5):700–16.

Cancer Screening in the Older Adult: Issues and Concerns

Melissa Craft, PhD, APRN, CNS, AOCN

KEYWORDS

- Cancer screening • Older adult • Issues • Decision making

KEY POINTS

- Recommendation for cancer screening in the older adult is based on multiple factors, which include evidence-based guidelines for screening, life expectancy and health status, risks and benefits, and individual values and wishes.
- The development of decision aids is helpful, but additional studies related to effective methods of communicating about individual recommendations for cancer screenings are needed.
- Clinicians need to look beyond their patient's chronologic age when advising about cancer screening.

Census projections indicate that the population of the world is aging and this trend will continue through the 21st century.[1] The incidence of cancer increases with age.[2] As the number of older adults increases, practitioners will be increasingly asked to give recommendations for cancer screening that include adults older than 75 years.[3] Although several practice guidelines give general recommendations for screening, many do not address specific issues of concern for older adults in this age range.[2] The issue is paradoxic; the rate of cancer increases in the older adult, it does not imply that routine cancer screening is recommended or even appropriate. Cancer screening in an older adult with serious comorbidities and limited life expectancy may cause more harm than projected good.[4,5] It is therefore important to consider the individual's current health, life expectancy, and understanding of the personal benefit of screening.[6] Having this conversation with patients may be difficult for some practitioners and may also be time consuming. In addition, patients may have a difficult time or even be resistant to having discussions about life expectancy and potential benefit based primarily on longevity.[7,8] In this article, the current recommendations for screening for breast cancer, cervical cancer, prostate cancer, and colon cancer in the older adult are presented. In addition to the current recommendations for screening, a model for incorporating current health and life expectancy is discussed,

Disclosures: None.
University of Oklahoma Health Sciences Center College of Nursing, 1100 North Stonewall Avenue, Room 420, Oklahoma City OK 73117, USA
E-mail address: Melissa-craft@ouhsc.edu

Nurs Clin N Am 49 (2014) 251–261
http://dx.doi.org/10.1016/j.cnur.2014.02.010
0029-6465/14/$ – see front matter © 2014 Elsevier Inc. All rights reserved.

as well as thoughts on how to present complex information in a usable, personalized format, by which to make decisions on cancer screenings.

POPULATION PREDICTIONS

According to the United Nations, the number of people older than 60 years in the world is expected to increase by 45% by the middle of the 21st century, more than tripling the current number, increasing from 841 million in 2013 to 3 billion in 2100. Even more impressive is the number of adults aged 80 years or older. This number is expected to increase almost 7-fold by 2100: 120 million in 2013 to 830 million in 2100. In developed countries, where cancer screening is more prevalent, life expectancy is projected to be 76 years of age by 2050 and 82 years by 2100, with 27% of the population expected to be 60 years and older.[9] The US Census Bureau predicts that those 85 years and older are expected to triple in the 21st century and the number of older adults will be 1 in 5 versus the current ratio of 1 in 7.[1] For practitioners, this situation means that about 20% of patients need information for screening decisions and a large proportion of those conversations need to include recommendations for the older adult, who may or may not have the current health or life expectancy needed to make cancer screening the best choice.

DECISION MAKING ABOUT CANCER SCREENING

Decisions about cancer screening take into consideration a patient's age, current health, and life expectancy.[10,11] Of these 3 criteria, many practitioners seem to primarily base their recommendations on age alone.[12,13] It is unclear whether practitioners routinely have conversations with their patients about the potential risks associated with screening, particularly because benefit/risk ratios change with diminished health and decreased life expectancy.[13,14]

Although the benefits and risks of screening vary based on the particular screening test, there are some general principles related to determining an individual's particular risk and benefit that apply to all of them. Walter, Covinsky and colleagues[4,6] and Bellury and colleagues[5] developed frameworks for decision making that incorporate 4 elements; up-to-date evidence-based practice guidelines, the patient's risk of dying based on life expectancy and comorbidities, benefits and risks of screening and the patient's preferences and values.

PRACTICE GUIDELINES

Using this framework can help the busy practitioner organize all the necessary steps to providing patient-focused care related to cancer screening decision making. The most current guidelines specific to stopping screening in the older adult for breast, cervical, colon, and prostate cancer are summarized (**Table 1**) from information from the American Cancer Society (ACS), the US Preventive Services Task Force (USPSTF), the American Geriatric Society, and the American Association of Family Physicians. These guidelines generally recommend that for breast cancer, a woman continue screening until the age of 75 years. Colon cancer screening begins at 50 years for average-risk individuals; cervical cancer screening can stop at 65 to 70 years in average-risk women who have previously been screened with no abnormal findings; prostate cancer screening with prostate-specific antigen is not recommended for average-risk men at any age. These recommendations are limited by the paucity of studies specifically targeting older adults and the inconsistency about when to stop screening. Cervical and prostate cancer recommendations are consistent across organizations; however, both breast and colon cancer have inconsistent recommendations regarding when to stop screening. The USPSTF carries the strongest stopping recommendations for both of these cancers, with the statement that there is no evidence that the benefits of mammography after 75 years outweigh the risks. Likewise, for colon cancer, the USPSTF recommends a hard stop of routine screening older than 75 years and complete stopping of screening older than 85 years. The ACS, on the other hand, has no stopping recommendation for colon cancer. This inconsistency in recommendations leads some agencies, like the American Association of Family Physicians and the American Geriatric Society, to emphasize the need to individualize recommendations to the specific patient using frameworks such as the one created by Walter and Covinsky (2001).[6] This framework weighs benefits and harms as 2 sides of a balance scale, in which the fulcrum consists of patient preferences that move from 1 side or the other to influence decisions about screening.

LIFE EXPECTANCY AND COMORBIDITY

The next step of the Walter and Covinsky framework is to consider the patient's life expectancy and health status. Clinicians have emphasized using evidence-based tools to assist the clinician in determining as best as possible the life expectancy for living cohorts to balance the risk and benefits of individual decisions.[6,25,26] Walter and Covinsky published an excellent tool that examines life expectancy per upper, middle and lower quartiles depending on the individual's comorbidities and where they fall similar to others in their age range.[6] Those individuals with the most comorbidities are in the lower quartile, whereas those with no comorbidities are in the upper quartile for life expectancy. Lee and colleagues[27] have developed a decision aid that includes life expectancy and current health, which is easy to use and available as an electronic mobile application to assist clinicians in individualizing their recommendations. This aid, Eprognosis.com, is also recommended by the National Comprehensive Cancer Network (NCCN) Clinical Practice Guidelines for Senior Adult Oncology.[28] As with any statistical tool based on population data, there are potential errors when applying to the individual, and therefore, the use of life expectancy calculators and decision aids continues to be recommended as only a piece of the assessment of risks and benefits for a particular screening recommendation and is not meant to replace clinical judgment.[3,29] However, these tools enable a busy practitioner to quickly assess issues known to increase the likelihood that a specific patient will not benefit from screening. For example, a woman who is 75 years old but has multiple comorbidities, does not live alone because of her functional status, and cannot manage her activities of daily living because of her cognitive functioning may truly have more risks associated with a decision to screen for breast or colon cancer than a healthy, independent 83-year-old. The consensus is that age alone is a poor tool to estimate individual risk versus benefits for screening.

BIOLOGY OF CANCER RELATED TO LIFE EXPECTANCY

Many patients, and some clinicians, struggle with understanding why life expectancy and health status are such important elements in the framework of screening decision making.[14,30] The rationale for the importance of predicting life expectancy is that the survival benefit from screening is not immediate. Multiple studies have shown that breast, colon, prostate, and cervical cancer survival curves do not start diverging from the screened versus unscreened until approximately 5 to 10 years after screening.[15–18] This situation is because the cancers found by routine screening of asymptomatic, average-risk individuals who have had negative previous screening

Table 1
Practice guidelines

	Breast	Colon	Cervical	Prostate
American Cancer Society	There is no specific upper age at which mammography screening should be discontinued. Rather, the decision to stop regular mammography screening should be individualized based on the potential benefits and risks of screening within the context of overall health status and estimated longevity. If a woman is in good health and would be a candidate for breast cancer treatment, she should continue to be screened with mammography. Life expectancy >5 y[2]	Average-risk adults should begin colorectal cancer screening at age 50 y. No recommendation for stopping[2]	Women >65 y who have had regular cervical cancer testing with normal results should not be tested for cervical cancer[2]	Because prostate cancer often grows slowly, men without symptoms of prostate cancer who do not have a 10-y life expectancy should not be offered testing, because they are not likely to benefit. Overall health status, and not age alone, is important when making decisions about screening[2]

US Preventive Services Task Force	For screening mammography in women ≥75 y, evidence is lacking and the balance of benefits and harms cannot be determined[15]	Adults age 76-85 y do not screen routinely. Adults >85 y do not screen. The likelihood that detection and early intervention yield a mortality benefit declines after age 75 y, because of the long average time between adenoma development and cancer diagnosis[16]	Recommends against screening for cervical cancer in women >65 y who have had adequate previous screening and are not otherwise at high risk for cervical cancer[17]	Do not use prostate-specific antigen–based screening for prostate cancer[18]
American Geriatric Society	May continue in women with life expectancy >5 y[19]	Screen all adults >50 y. Persons too frail to undergo colonoscopy and persons with short life expectancy (3–5 y) should not be screened[20]	There is little evidence for or against screening women beyond age 70 y who have been regularly screened in previous years[21]	No recommendation
American Association of Family Physicians	Information is lacking about the effectiveness of screening in women ≥75 y. The decision to screen women in this age group should be individualized, keeping the patient's life expectancy, functional status, and goals in mind[22]	Continue screening until 75 y[23]	Recommends against screening for cervical cancer in women >65 y who have had adequate previous screening and are not otherwise at risk for cervical cancer[24]	Recommends against prostate-specific antigen–based screening for prostate cancer[25]

are at an early stage.[14] This is the founding principle of an ideal screening test.[30] However, this situation means that if the patient has been regularly screened, is not high risk and is not symptomatic, the natural history of the cancer is that it takes approximately 5 to 10 years to develop to the point at which it poses a mortality risk for the patient. If the mortality curves occurred earlier, it would indicate that the cancer was further along in its natural history than predicted and theoretically should have been found in an earlier screening, when treatment would have altered the survivability of the cancer. As Lee and colleagues[27] report, the time lag to benefit exposes individuals to immediate risks of screening, with potentially little chance to benefit if their life expectancy is less than the time lag to benefit. Lee and colleagues[27] conducted a survival meta-analysis for breast and colon cancer, which showed that it takes 4.8 years before 1 death from colon cancer was prevented for 5000 people screened and 10.3 years before 1 death was prevented for 1000 people screened. In breast cancer, these investigators found 3 years elapsed before 1 death was prevented for 5000 women screened and 10.7 years before 1 death was prevented per 1000 women screened. Schonberg and colleagues[31] reviewed data from a national health interview and found that most women older than 80 years had a life expectancy of less than 10 years, yet more than half were still receiving routine mammography. Others have corroborated this finding and suggested that current screening recommendations by practitioners are still predominantly driven by age and not by comorbidity.[10,32] Part of the difficulty in individualizing screening recommendations based on patient life expectancy and health status is the sheer complexity of this information, with the number of factors that have to be weighed.[8,33,34] However, other barriers for both the practitioner and the patient in using life expectancy and health status as a part of the decision making is the expectations for screening. Many patients derive other benefits from screening (or believe they do) than a survival benefit. Research shows that most people overestimate their risk of cancer, and many associate screening with longevity and better care.[31] The generation of older adults confronting this decision making dilemma have come to age in a society that has progressively promoted being proactive with health screenings. This ingrained behavior may be associated with staying alive even when other comorbid conditions alter the benefit that can be expected at an individual level in a standard-risk person. Lewis and colleagues[8] found that most residents older than 70 years living in long-term care communities did not believe that life expectancy was important for decisions about screening, and almost half preferred not to talk about life expectancy. Although important to the individualized decision making process for screening recommendations, it is apparent that life expectancy and health status are not being used fully, and more research on useful tools, methods of discussing and explaining the lag time of screening in proportion to life expectancy, and acceptance of such discussions by providers and patients is needed.

RISKS AND BENEFITS OF CANCER SCREENING

The need to consider life expectancy and health status to make a decision about screening is predicated on the fact that screening carries potential risks as well as benefits. Many risks are apparent and immediate, because they relate to the screening test itself. Because prostate cancer and cervical cancer screening is consistently not recommended in the older adult, this discussion focuses on risks and benefits for colon and breast cancer screening. **Table 2** is a synopsis of the risks and benefits of the screening itself, subsequent tests and procedures related to a positive screen, plus burdens related to screening, such as transportation issues and costs.

Table 2
Risks, benefits, and burdens of breast and colon cancer screening

Cancer	Benefits of Screening	Risks of Screening	Risks of Additional Procedures Related to Screening	Burdens of Screening
Breast	Identification of early stage breast cancer	Pain related to mammogram (worsened in patients with mobility issues, particularly shoulder mobility, because of positioning) Embarrassment related to mammogram[19]	Infection, bruising, and swelling from biopsy site	Securing transportation Cost of initial screening and subsequent procedures
Colon	Identification of early stage colon cancer	Pain related to sigmoidoscopy or colonoscopy Potential bowel perforation Potential bleeding Cardiopulmonary events (Whitlock from slides) Embarrassment/ offensiveness of procedure[35]	Bleeding from biopsies Potential additional tests such as computed tomography with contrast dye, which may be renal toxic	Securing transportation Cost of initial screening and subsequent procedures

Other risks include the psychological burden of experiencing a false-positive screening test. Many patients who have a positive result from a screening test become anxious about the result, and subsequent tests that are ordered.[12] The waiting period between positive screen and additional testing can be days to weeks and may include several procedures. Many patients are overwhelmed by the uncertainty of their diagnosis during this time and report higher levels of anxiety and depression even after they are determined not to have cancer.[36] This situation may be magnified in those individuals who have cognitive or sensory problems, which may make these tests and follow-up procedures more difficult, painful, or frightening.[37]

In addition, practitioners may not consider the risks of the treatments that would be recommended if the patient is found to have a cancer. The use of a comprehensive geriatric assessment (CGA) is recommended by the Clinical Practice Guidelines in Senior Adult Oncology from the NCCN[28] when initially evaluating a newly diagnosed older adult patient who has cancer. Completing this assessment as part of the screening decision making might help identify those patients who have functional decline that may affect their ability to cope with cancer treatment if a cancer is diagnosed.[5] Functional status is a key component of overall health among older patients who have cancer and has been shown to be a predictor for outcomes.[7] Koroukian[38] found that the presence of 2 or more geriatric syndromes was associated with unfavorable survival outcomes, and Kowdley and colleagues[30] reported the risks of surgery in the elderly and recommend strongly that older adult patients who have cancer and are undergoing surgery be assessed first with the CGA. Because the weighing of multiple pieces of information can be overwhelming and determining life expectancy for the individual may be difficult, clinicians may find that incorporating the CGA in their patients who may not be clearly in the lowest quartile or the highest quartile of life expectancy can help them make a screening recommendation. This situation may be especially true if a clinician thinks a patient would not have more risk than benefit from the screening test but can see a potential for more risk than benefit for the treatment of the cancer if found.

INDIVIDUAL WISHES AND BELIEFS

Treating a cancer once found is generally an ethical imperative. An analogous ethical treatment dilemma is taking a patient off a ventilator once they have been placed on it. The purpose of advanced directives is to give an individual the opportunity to have input into a significant decision while they still can and avoid having to undo something that increases individual and family burdens.[39] Likewise, the purpose of considering a patient's wishes and values before making a recommendation for screening is to acknowledge that one of the biggest risks of screening for cancer in an older adult with limited life expectancy is that a cancer is found that might be described as inconsequential disease.[6] It is difficult to imagine that a cancer could be considered inconsequential, but the definition of this is that it is a cancer that would never have progressed enough to affect patient survival during the patient's lifetime.[14] Therefore, the cancer is diagnosed and treatment is usually initiated, with all of its consequences, both physical and psychological, but the cancer would never have killed the patient during their lifetime or affected their quality of life. One of the difficulties in evaluating this issue is that the lag time for benefit of screening is based on survival of the cancer; however, there are cancer symptoms that may seriously affect a patient's quality of life.[27] The lag time to development of those symptoms certainly may be shorter than death, and benefits might be seen in finding a cancer early enough to avoid some of those symptoms, for example, if a breast cancer is detected early enough to allow a simple surgical procedure such as partial mastectomy versus later diagnosis when the cancer presents as a fungating mass that is inoperable and causes pain, infection, and embarrassment. Theoretically, the amount of time it takes to naturally progress to that advanced stage is longer than the patient's life expectancy, but the uncertainty of that prediction is the crux of how difficult these recommendations are. The alternative to this example is a very early stage breast cancer, such as ductal carcinoma in situ (DCIS), which biologically progresses to invasive breast cancer less than 50% of the time.[2] If a woman is diagnosed with this cancer and receives surgery to remove the tissue of concern, develops an infection, undergoes multiple rounds of antibiotics, perhaps even having to pack the wound followed by potential chronic pain, then she has not had an improved quality of life because of early diagnosis of breast cancer. The overdiagnosis of cancer usually leads to overtreatment.[16] Slow-growing and biologically less aggressive cancers make up the bulk of inconsequential disease; however, they carry significant consequences for the patient, both physically and psychologically, once diagnosed. The way to avoid diagnosing these cancers, leading to subsequent decision making regarding treatment, is to not screen.

TO SCREEN OR NOT TO SCREEN

Without a crystal ball, there is no way to know exactly how all the elements of Walter and Covinsky's model will work for the individual in the present and in the future. What is becoming clearer is that the recommendation for cancer screening in the older adult is based on multiple factors, which include evidence-based guidelines for screening, life expectancy and health status, risks and benefits, and individual values and wishes. Weighing all of these factors together and communicating complex information to the patient can be difficult and time consuming. The development of decision aids is helpful, but additional studies related to effective methods of communicating about this issue are needed. In the meantime, clinicians need to look beyond their patient's chronologic age when advising about cancer screening. Although this may be a difficult task, it is important and may not be as black and white as a clinician (or patient) initially thinks. The goal is that those who have the greatest benefit from screening are screened the most and those who have the least benefit are at least involved in an informed discussion about not screening. Both the individual and the greater good is served when resources are used appropriately.

REFERENCES

1. US Census Bureau. US Census Bureau projections show a slower growing, older, more diverse nation a half century from now. 2012. Available at: http://www.census.gov/population/projections/data/national/2012/pressreleases.html. Accessed September 4, 2013.
2. Smith RA, Brooks D, Cokkinides V, et al. Cancer screening in the United States, 2013: a review of current American Cancer Society guidelines, current issues in cancer screening, and new guidance on cervical cancer screening and lung cancer screening. CA Cancer J Clin 2013;63(2):88–105.
3. Yourman LC, Lee SJ, Schonberg MA, et al. Prognostic indices for older adults: a systematic review. JAMA 2012;307(2):182–92.
4. Walter LC, Eng C, Covinsky KE. Screening mammography for frail older women. J Gen Intern Med 2001;16(11):779–84.
5. Bellury LM, Ellington L, Beck SL, et al. Elderly cancer survivorship: an integrative review and conceptual framework. Eur J Oncol Nurs 2011;15(3):233–42.
6. Walter LC, Covinsky KE. Cancer screening in elderly patients: a framework for individualized decision making. JAMA 2001;285(21):2750–6.
7. Resnick B. Health promotion practices of older adults: testing an individualized approach. J Clin Nurs 2003;12(1):46–55 [discussion: 56].
8. Lewis CL, Kistler CE, Amick HR, et al. Older adults' attitudes about continuing cancer screening later in life: a pilot study interviewing residents of two continuing care communities. BMC Geriatr 2006;6:10.
9. United Nations. Department of Economic and Social Affairs: population division. 2013. Available at: http://www.un.org/en/development/desa/population/. Accessed August 21, 2013.
10. Walter LC, Lewis CL, Barton MB. Screening for colorectal, breast, and cervical cancer in the elderly: a review of the evidence. Am J Med 2005;118(10):1078–86.
11. Lee SJ, Lindquist K, Segal MR, et al. Development and validation of a prognostic index for 4-year mortality in older adults. JAMA 2006;295(7):801–8.
12. Boyd CM, Darer J, Boult C, et al. Clinical practice guidelines and quality of care for older patients with multiple comorbid diseases: implications for pay for performance. JAMA 2005;294(6):716–24.
13. Albert RH, Clark MM. Cancer screening in the older patient. Am Fam Physician 2008;78(12):1369–74.
14. Walter LC. Cancer screening in older adults. In: Hurria A, Balducci L, editors. Geriatric oncology. New York: Springer Science+Business Media, LLC; 2009. p. 47–70.
15. US Preventive Services Task Force. Screening for breast cancer. 2010. Available at: http://www.uspreventiveservicestaskforce.org/uspstf/uspsbrca.htm. Accessed July 12, 2013.

16. US Preventive Services Task Force. Screening for colon cancer. 2009. Available at: http://www.uspreventiveservicestaskforce.org/uspstf/uspscolo.htm. Accessed July 12, 2013.

17. US Preventive Services Task Force. Screening for cervical cancer. 2012. Available at: http://www.uspreventiveservicestaskforce.org/uspstf/uspscerv.htm. Accessed July 12, 2013.

18. US Preventive Services Task Force. Screening for prostate cancer. 2012. Available at: http://www.uspreventiveservicestaskforce.org/prostatecancerscreening.htm. Accessed July 12, 2013.

19. American Geriatrics Society Clinical Practice Committee. Breast cancer screening in older women. J Am Geriatr Soc 2000;48(7):842–4.

20. US Preventive Services Task Force. Colon cancer screening (USPSTF recommendation). J Am Geriatr Soc 2000;48:333–5.

21. American Geriatrics Society. Screening for cervical cancer in older women. J Am Geriatr Soc 2001;49:655–7.

22. American Academy of Family Physicians. Breast cancer screening update. 2013. Available at: https://secure.aafp.org/login/. Accessed August 27, 2013.

23. American Academy of Family Physicians. Colon cancer screening. 2008. Available at: http://www.aafp.org/afp/2008/1215/p1393.html. Accessed August 27, 2013.

24. American Academy of Family Physicians. Cervical cancer. 2012. Available at: http://www.aafp.org/patient-care/clinical-recommendations/all/cervical-cancer.html. Accessed August 27, 2013.

25. American Academy of Family Physicians. Prostate cancer. 2012. Available at: http://www.aafp.org/patient-care/clinical-recommendations/all/prostate-cancer.html. Accessed August 27, 2013.

26. Rodin MB. Estimating life expectancy. Presented at the American Geriatrics Society Annual Science Meeting. Seattle, May 3, 2012.

27. Lee SJ, Boscardin WJ, Stijacic-Cenzer I, et al. Time lag to benefit after screening for breast and colorectal cancer: meta-analysis of survival data from the United States, Sweden, United Kingdom, and Denmark. BMJ 2013;346:e8441.

28. National Comprehensive Cancer Network. Clinical practice guidelines: senior adult oncology. 2013. Available at: http://www.nccn.org/professionals/physician_gls/f_guidelines.asp-age. Accessed August 28, 2013.

29. Schonberg MA. Decision aids. The answer we've been looking for? Presented at the American Geriatrics Society Annual Science meeting. Grapevine, May 4, 2013.

30. Kowdley GC, Merchant N, Richardson JP, et al. Cancer surgery in the elderly. ScientificWorldJournal 2012;2012:303852.

31. Schonberg MA, McCarthy EP, Davis RB, et al. Breast cancer screening in women aged 80 and older: results from a national survey. J Am Geriatr Soc 2004;52(10):1688–95.

32. Walter LC. Framework for screening decision making. Presented at the American Geriatrics Society Annual Science Meeting. Grapevine, May 4, 2013.

33. Klabunde CN, Frame PS, Meadow A, et al. A national survey of primary care physicians' colorectal cancer screening recommendations and practices. Prev Med 2003;36:352–62.

34. Lewis CL, Griffith J, Pignone MP, et al. Physicians' decisions about continuing or stopping colon cancer screening in the elderly: a qualitative study. J Gen Intern Med 2009;24(7):816–21.

35. Beeker C, Kraft JM, Southwell BG, et al. Colorectal cancer screening in older men and women: qualitative research findings and implications for intervention. J Community Health 2000;25(3):263–78.

36. Deane KA, Degner LF. Information needs, uncertainty, and anxiety in women who had a breast biopsy with benign outcome. Cancer Nurs 1998;21(2):117–26.

37. Sox HC. Screening for disease in older people. J Gen Intern Med 1998;13(6): 424–5.

38. Koroukian SM. Assessment and interpretation of comorbidity burden in older adults with cancer. J Am Geriatr Soc 2009;57(Suppl 2):S275–8.

39. Hackler C. Advance directives and the refusal of treatment. Med Law 1989;7(5): 457–65.

Index

Note: Page numbers of article titles are in **boldface** type.

Nurs Clin N Am 49 (2014) 263–268
http://dx.doi.org/10.1016/S0029-6465(14)00025-5
0029-6465/14/$ – see front matter © 2014 Elsevier Inc. All rights reserved.

Moving?

Make sure your subscription moves with you!

To notify us of your new address, find your **Clinics Account Number** (located on your mailing label above your name), and contact customer service at:

Email: journalscustomerservice-usa@elsevier.com

800-654-2452 (subscribers in the U.S. & Canada)
314-447-8871 (subscribers outside of the U.S. & Canada)

Fax number: 314-447-8029

Elsevier Health Sciences Division
Subscription Customer Service
3251 Riverport Lane
Maryland Heights, MO 63043

*To ensure uninterrupted delivery of your subscription, please notify us at least 4 weeks in advance of move.